The Fat Genes Are Talking

A Woman's Confrontations with Weight-Loss Shenanigans

LaTonya Carmouché

NOAH'S ARK PUBLISHING, LLC.

The Fat Genes Are Talking

A Woman's Confrontations with Weight-Loss Shenanigans

LaTonya Carmouché

The Fat Genes Are Talking

ISBN 978-0-692-12997-5

Noah's Ark Publishing
Service 8549 Wilshire Blvd.,
Suite 1442
Beverly Hills, CA 90211
www.LAVALDREAMS.com
noahsarkpublishing@gmail.com
Lavaldreams / Noah's Ark Publishing Service LLC

Formatted by Jenine May, President Kingdom Scribes

Cover graphics by Donnie L. Hill, CEO Donnie Graphics

Photograph by Sir Jones @sirjonesmedia

Table of Contents

Dedication	7
Acknowledgements	9
Introduction	11
Chapter One - Growing Up	17
Chapter Two - The Plot of the Fat Genes	41
Chapter Three - Losing Control	55
Chapter Four - May I Take Your Order	71
Chapter Five - The ~~Steaks~~ Stakes Are Higher	95
Chapter Six - The Six-Foot Candy Bar	103
Chapter Seven - Flashbacks of the Sabotage - The Real Aha Moment	119
Chapter Eight - Loser Mentality - Finding My Worth	135
Chapter Nine - In Tune with My Body Needs	141

DEDICATION

Charity, inside and out, you are breathtakingly beautiful. Your existence has taught me how to give and receive love from an unspeakable level. Your eyes remind me of God's incredible love. I stand in awe at your magnificence, tenacity for life, and innate wisdom. You have and continue to motivate me to reach limits I once only dreamt of. I strive for greatness not just for myself, but for you as well. I see you watching. I am grateful I have you to travel with during this wonderful experience called life. Our journey has just begun! ~ Mommy

ACKNOWLEDGEMENTS

First and foremost, I have to acknowledge my savior, Jesus Christ. From my health to my wealth, all that I am, I owe to Him. Thank you, God, for loving me and giving me grace, patience, mercy and guidance as I continually learn to grow in You.

To my loving and amazing parents, Jesse and Doreatha Carmouche. Having parents such as yourselves has helped mold me into the woman I am today. For that I am grateful. Your love and support mean the world to me. Thank you.

My siblings and in-loves, Jesse, Shelly, Valencia, Demetria "Mimi", Joaquin, and Kristina, you guys are the best! It feels like the years have lessened the gaps, no more "bigs", "smalls" and me, now it is just us. As adults we know how to work together as a unit and get things done. Mimi and Joaquin, you two are my right and left arms, you are my rock stars. Thank you all for supporting me. The love we have for one another is truly God, let's forever keep this connection.

My tribe of nieces and nephews: This book started off as a funny comic for me to share with you. I wanted you to have something from your TT that will always make you laugh. It turned into therapy for me. Thank you for being my influence to write. I love you all!

My superstar TCPR clients: Thank you all for believing in me, trusting in me and understanding when I had to slow down a bit to focus on my family and myself. The best is yet to come for all of us. I still have your back!

My listening team/extended family: Charity, Myra, Phala, Ben, Anne, Joshua, Antracia, Aalure, Jacquelyn, Rochelle, Justin, Xavier, Jay, Tyrone, Brandon, Desreta, and Melvin, from the beginning of this project until the end, you allowed me to share bits with you and gave me honest feedback and encouragement. I appreciate you!

I will not begin to list friends because I may leave someone out, just know if you have my personal number and I answer your calls after 10 p.m., I love you and appreciate the role you play in my life.

LaVal Belle and Noah's Ark Publishing, you believed in me from the start. I will forever be thankful. Now let's make this a bestseller.

INTRODUCTION

Doesn't it feel good to feel like you have power, you are in control and you are carefree? That is how food made me feel at times when it seemed as if I had no control over anything around me. It was the only thing that I felt I could control. I could eat what I wanted pretty much when I wanted it. All of the chips, candy, hamburgers, pizza, Rock Star energy drinks, French fries, oh my gosh, especially the French fries, they all delivered immediate satisfaction and I unknowingly lost control. In fact, it was as if my control were being controlled by a force, little aliens that invaded my mind and body.

These little aliens seem so real, I used my imagination to give them a name. I call them Fat Genes, FGs for short. The influence and energy the FGs give are intense. They are deceitful, sneaky and sly. A force to be reckoned with. The FGs talk to one another and they would use anything they could to overtake me and wipe me off the face of this Earth.

Everyday stresses were triggers for me to eat. The Los Angeles traffic, people who drive as if they are in a rush to go nowhere influenced me to keep an energy drink in the car so I could have the strength to focus on the road-raged maniacs while remaining sane and calm. Reporting to the boss who demands more than an 8-hour shift can handle, being given work that is clearly out of my scope but being asked to handle it without being given the proper tools or resources to accomplish an end-goal, which forced me to be creative, get the job done but not jeopardize my employment… I snacked on junk all day at my desk to help me tolerate working with people who seem to have been hired solely based on looks or their ability to speak another language but had no real clue on how to handle work or conduct themselves in a professional manner.

Being a single mother, being responsible to make sure food is in the house, my daughter has proper clothes for the weather, gas in the vehicle, house is clean, homework is done, bills are paid, student loans attended to, wanting to be a homeowner but living from paycheck to paycheck so how can I save?

Losing the feeling that your parents are immortals because you are watching them age and slow down daily. Seeing children growing up and having to deal with other children who missed out on home training. Feeling stuck in a position at work because I am either overqualified with my Master's degree or don't have enough experience. Just a bunch of stuff that made me want to eat junk food, if I was hungry or not.

Those triggers gave me the false belief that I was powerless and had no control. That was the very thing that opened the door to the Fat Genes to overtake my mind and body. I gained 100 pounds and allowed myself to adjust to the additional weight for years, until I had to face the reality that the excess weight was killing me. I started an all-out war, an internal battle of me fighting for my life and getting rid of the 100 pounds that I see as individual Fat Genes working together to destroy me. They must be killed one by one before they kill me.

I believe being healthy is very important. I also believe laughing at yourself is just as important. This book started off as a joke. It was a creative way to excuse my lack of self-discipline. I was creating characteristics for my Fat Gene frienemies and using my imagination to give them personalities to justify me being overweight in my own humorous way. Then, I had a serious reality check that made me face what was slowly killing me. Obviously, Fat Genes do not talk, nor are they beings that can sabotage your weight loss. For me, they were just a fun excuse to justify me not loving myself as I should. I allowed myself to be content with constantly starting the path to health and detouring, starting and detouring.

It is amazing how I went so long not realizing that it is not being selfish to love me, to take time for myself and appreciate my temple. It was not until a wonderful and brilliant friend of mine told me I wouldn't feel guilty if I realized the importance of self-first and stopped calling it selfish. The way he said it sunk in and caused me to wake up and own my truth. When I chose to be real with myself I accepted that I did not have any real reasons for my self-induced, well-hidden unhappiness and it was totally up to me to make a change.

This book is a journey through my up-and-down battles with becoming healthy and getting to a healthy weight. My desire is for my story not only to entertain, I want readers to laugh because they can relate to my weight-loss shenanigans and I hope it is an eye opener for those who have never struggled with weight and do not understand how someone would "allow" themselves to be unhealthy.

Most of all I want readers to know that whether it is weight, alcohol, drugs, sex, work, television, a pet, or a loved one, most of us have some sort of vice or addiction that is distracting us from being our best self, from being who God ordained us to be.

We can slowly drift away and lose focus from our life's purpose, or we may discover our purpose and have it cut short or, worse, miss our purpose altogether, if we don't be honest with ourselves, value ourselves and find a life balance that allows us to realize our purpose and finish the mission we were sent to Earth to complete.

We all have something we struggle with and we all have the choice to tackle our vice or allow distractions, large or small, have power over us. For years I allowed distractions to have power over me. Well, the buck finally stopped. No more distractions for me. Take a look around, I am not the only one who was "gifted" with Fat Genes. Some of us were born with them, some of us invited them into to our bodies, some of us had them come along uninvitingly because of medications, physical accidents, etc. The point is, I am not the only one who has a battle with Fat Genes, I am just going to be one of the few that will expose them for who they are. They are little demons that invade our thought process and convince us that everything is out of our control.

Have you noticed the growing rate of childhood obesity, the rising number of young adult obesity? These imaginary Fat Genes are killing us at 30, 40 and 50 years of age. I started writing this book seven years ago, (time flies!). While rereading the only two paragraphs that I had written, I was ashamed at how I unknowingly discredited the good I was doing at ridding all the unwanted FGs and fell for the mental trap that these Fat Genes set up for me. I gave my power away and allowed them to come back and bring ten extra friends with them.

I know now that this is an everyday mindset, it is not just enough to say I will change, I have to take action and purposely decide every minute of the day not to allow the FGs to rule my life. Travel with me on this journey to health as I have to combat and fight the Fat Genes daily! Let the shenanigans begin…

Chapter One

Growing Up

Do you believe the position you hold in your family sort of dictates your personality and your position in life? I do. I am a middle child, I have two older siblings, Jesse and Valencia, who are 5 and 7 years older than I am. Then I have two younger siblings, Demetria and Joaquin, who are 7 and 9 years younger than I am. With them each being two years apart from a sibling, they had each other to grow up with. Whereas, with me, I was too young to run with the "bigs" and too old to play with the "smalls", so I existed in a category by myself.

I was smack dead in the middle. There were times when I felt alone or unseen because, perhaps the "bigs" were out with friends and the "smalls" were being entertained and nurtured by our mother. Our father was mostly at work, he was the sole provider for a family of seven, so working was pretty much the bulk of his day. I never complained about my position or feeling of loneliness because I learned to make it work and ultimately came to appreciate my space. This allowed me to develop independence and creative ways to entertain myself, mostly with books, writing, and music.

I was able to adapt to my lifestyle, the feelings of loneliness and feeling invisible because I made it work. I guess this was the beginning of the nurturing of my fat genes. They gave me internal and mental company when I was feeling lonely and unseen. I catered to them and them to me. We made it work until it didn't.

Physically, I was not born alone. I believe when a newborn comes into this world he or she does not come alone. Some people believe they come with guardian angels, spirits of loves ones that have passed, special gifts that will attribute to world-changing events, and in my case Fat Genes!!

On November 21, 1971, my two loving parents introduced me, a 7-pound, 1-ounce baby girl name LaTonya Carmouche, to the world. I was born at General Hospital in Los Angeles, CA. My niece Aalure gave me the nickname TT and it just stuck. I am called TT by family, friends, and anyone that I feel comfortable around is welcomed to call me TT.

To me, TT is the fun, loving, cool, easygoing, hip person everyone wants to be around. I just had to learn that being fun, loving, cool, easygoing is not OK for everyone, everything, or every situation.

I left the hospital a normal, healthy child. My parents didn't notice I was leaving with a "gift", the doctors could not detect it, in fact it took me years to acknowledge and accept the "gift" I came home with almost forty years earlier. My gift was 100 Fat Genes that would act as the lover of my life and eventually become 100 pounds and in due course turn out to be one of my worst nightmares.

My father is a quiet but strong, brilliant, handsome Afro-American man. He stands 5-feet-11 inches tall and always had a slender build with broad shoulders. He is best known for his tremendous work ethic. He is always working. If not at a corporation job, he was repairing somebody's furniture in our garage or working on somebody's car in our driveway. My father has God-given intelligence. He didn't get much schooling but he can teach a lot of people valuable life lessons.

My father can tell time by looking at the sun or moon. He can make a car run on a wire hanger and a few screws, he can look at a room and tell you exactly how many cans of paint you would need to paint it, and if you ever try to tell him a lie, he will look at you and instantly say, I don't believe it. His intelligence and instincts cannot be found in a book. He is the smartest man I know.

My mom is one of the most beautiful women I have ever seen. She stands 5-feet tall, flawless skin, she used to dye her hair an auburn honey blonde, gorgeous big eyes and a smile that still lights up a room. Unlike my dad, my mom talks a lot. She has a gentle, angelic voice that comforts listeners when she speaks and she always has something wise to say.

She is creative in her own right, she always kept our house looking like a home by using some sort of contraption she found at the local store. She is an amazing cook. She was known around the neighborhood as "Angel" because of her Christ-like demeanor.

When I was a baby, maybe 3 or 4, I remember my father would drive the "bigs" and me to my grandmother's house on 111th Street in Los Angeles before he went to his day job. My grandmother's house was a small, one-story home that always smelled like delicious food. We were never allowed to enter from the front door, everyone knew to drive or walk to the back and knock on that door. Although my grandmother always sat in the front of the house, she demanded we enter through the back and she preferred to walk all the way to the back of the house to open the door and allow us to come inside.

Entering into the back room was like entering into a multipurpose room. There was a full-size bed, a sewing machine sitting on a table, a huge stereo that no one ever played music on, an office desk covered with office supplies, a dresser filled with extra clothing, a washing machine, dryer, Arrowhead water cooler, a television and a small bathroom.

Almost everything you needed in a house was located in this one room. What I remember most about this room was a small radio that stayed on 24 hours a day, tuned to KEARTH 101 radio station. The carpet throughout the house was covered in plastic runners that had these ribbed, pointy grips at the bottom. If you ever stepped on the backside of the runner barefoot, it felt like needles were stabbing your foot. The hallway was wall papered with white paper that had black velvet shapes all over it. I liked rubbing my hand across the velvet as I walked down the hallway to the front of the house.

A few steps down the hall on the left was my grandmother's room. It was a tiny room with a big bed, a makeup table, and a chair. I never walked past my grandmother's room and saw an unmade bed. On her makeup table she always kept a hair brush, comb, bottle of pink Oil of Olay, one tube of Revlon lipstick, Coty face powder, lotion and a bottle of perfume.

Across from her room was another room with twin-size beds, a baby crib, a huge bookcase filled with Encyclopedias, dictionaries and random yearbooks from mother and aunts' school days. This was the go-to room for naps. Whoever was sleepy could go lay in here. Even at the age of 3 or 4, I remember I was always put in the baby crib. A few steps farther down the hall and just before the front door was a decent-sized living room and the kitchen.

The living room had two small sofas covered in plastic to match the plastic-covered floors, a large television, a table that could spin around and hold albums. All of the slots for the albums were filled but for some reason it seemed like the Johnny Mathis and Chicago albums stayed turned toward the front, as if having them displayed offered a "fancy" touch to the decor.

By the television there was a candy dish that always had butterscotch or peppermint treats. On certain days the dish would be filled with Andes chocolate mint candies. Normally, I could help myself to a butterscotch or peppermint, no questions asked. However, if I helped myself to an Andes chocolate, it was obvious someone had been in her "expensive" candy and everyone present would be asked, "Who been in the candy dish?"

On these days, I opted out of treating myself to the candy dish. The kitchen was connected to the living room. There was a sliding partition that could separate the two rooms, but no one ever used the partition. The living room and kitchen was like one humongous room. The kitchen was small and basic. There was a table, chairs, stove, refrigerator, and a sink with a mirror over it. Although this was the room with the least details, it was the room where the most love was felt.

Even with the table clear and nothing on the stove except a teapot, there was a presence that engulfed me with tremendous love whenever I stepped foot on the tile floor. I don't know if it is because the kitchen was the room my grandmother loved or if it was because the kitchen was the room where she cooked our food with so much love. The passion seeped from her pores and filled the air. Whatever the reason, the kitchen was the best room in the house and it was the room I could always find grandmother in.

We called my grandmother Muh. She was another one of the most beautiful women I have ever seen. She would always wear her hair in two, long and silky ponytails, her skin was flawless, she stood 5-feet-1 but seemed like a giant to me. She always smelled like Jergen's cherry almond lotion and pink Oil of Olay. She didn't speak much, but when she did speak it was with authority and certainty.

Whether it was her telling me, "Tonya, you are going to go far in life. Stay exactly who you are and mark my word. I see your greatness", or telling me "Keep acting up and I will grab you with my cane and bust your behind wide open", she was sincere and I believed every word she said.

I remember her mostly sitting at her kitchen table either preparing something to eat for all of the grandchildren she was caring for or playing solitaire. She loved to watch soap operas and game shows, she would always have one or the other programs blasting loud in the living room while she sat at the kitchen table watching from across the room.

The "bigs" and I weren't the only ones being dropped off. My aunts or uncles would drop my cousins off to Muh's house on their way to work as well. This would be around 7 a.m. every weekday morning. We would come in and Muh would fix us breakfast. I hated the days she would prepare chocolate Malt O' Meal because one of my cousins would always stuff their mouth then look at me and open their mouth showing the chewed up food to make me gag. I hate the site of mushy or chewed up food. There was on an average eleven of us at breakfast and they would all laugh at me. Muh would yell, "Tonya Ranette, stop being silly at the table and eat your breakfast!"

So now I am grossed out, crying and was being forced to eat this nasty looking bowl of blob while holding the image of all of the mush in someone else's mouth. Muh did not believe in wasting food, she did not care if I was crying or gagging. If she prepared it, I was going to eat it. I don't think I ever told her the reason I was acting up at the table. I am sure she would have done something, but rather than snitching, I learned to adapt.

Around 8 a.m. each day, my aunt would take the older seven grandchildren to school, leaving me and my three cousins alone with Muh. The cousins I stayed with daily were Michael, Lamont, and Sean. Michael and Lamont are brothers, they are a year apart and they were bad as heck. As soon as it was down to the four of us they would manage to get out of my grandmother's sight and find trouble.

Sean was like me. He was the baby in his family and his two older brothers were 9 and 10 years older than him, so he understood me and my feelings of being lonely but not alone. Like me, Sean did not like trouble, we were for the most part obedient and we found ways to entertain one another. Muh didn't care too much for us playing outside, I guess she didn't feel it was safe.

We certainly could never play in the front yard, out of her fear of someone from the local gang trying to grab us or something. Muh would tell us to go find something to do while she cleaned up the kitchen and started preparing the next meal. Sean and I would go to the back room to play Uno, make up funny stories, pretend we were a store owner and customers, tell jokes or watch cartoons, innocent things.

Meanwhile, Michael and Lamont would sneak outside to run up and down the street. If they weren't outside they were inside breaking something. They stayed in trouble and although Sean and I were behaving, we would all get in trouble when Michael and Lamont got caught. Muh would tell us we are family and we have to look out for one another. We should not sit idle and watch our cousins make mistakes. They got in trouble for being bad and we got in trouble for not stopping them.

It was never harsh trouble, we would just have to sit in the room in silence until she felt it was long enough. Sean would cry and cry, pleading it wasn't fair that we had to stop what we were doing to sit in silence with the bad boys. I on the other hand didn't care, I adapted to the silence and the punishment.

When I turned five, I was enrolled into kindergarten at 107th Street School in Los Angeles. This year stands out to me because not only did I get to go to school like the "bigs", but my mother was the teacher's aide for my class! I remember her driving me to school, and as she was driving she would hold my hand and sing, "LaTonya, LaTonya, mommy's little baby, I love you so and I won't let you go because you are mommy's baby."

It was our very own special time, I had my mom all to myself. She was able to see just me without having to blur her vision by also looking at my older brother or sister. She saw only me. The morning 20-30 minute drive meant the world to me, I felt special. When we got to school, of course I had to share her again with the other students, but that drive was a great way to start my day. We would walk in class and immediately she would have to lose focus on me because students would be calling her name.

In class, she told me to call her Mrs. Carmouche, not mom, because other kids would be jealous. That made me feel like one of them, and just like at home, I was just there, no one spectacular, just one of some. I didn't complain and I followed the rule, I adapted. I got my second chance to feel outstanding because I got to be seen with mom, or rather, Mrs. Carmouche, at lunch time.

We ate different lunches everyday but my favorite was corn dogs and tater tots. I would sit across from her on the lunch benches and feel like I was royalty. I would look at all of the other kids and think, I am the luckiest one here. My mom is here and she is eating lunch with just me! After lunch, I would go play on the playground with the other kids, and she would go back to the classroom but I was emotionally full for the day. I had all of my mother's attention for a brief time and it left me feeling extra special for the rest of the school day.

My summers at this time was mostly spent at Muh's house. I still hung with Sean, except now we were allowed to be outside because all of the "bigs" would be there. My cousins who are up to nine years older than me would want to go outside so Muh felt it was a littler safer for us younger kids to run free because she knew we were all trained to look out for one another.

During the summer, the male "bigs" were Eric, Kevin, Cammie, Byron and my brother Jesse. The female "bigs" were my cousin Deborah and my sister Valencia. The "smalls" were my barely older cousins, Michael, Lamont and my younger cousin Sean. We would go outside after breakfast and the "bigs" would throw footballs or play some other sport. Or they would stand around and talk as if they had some grown-up stuff to discuss. Michael and Lamont continued to find trouble while Sean and I played basketball or at least threw a basketball at the hoop. After a few hours, Muh would call us in to wash up for lunch.

Muh would literally sit at the table with two new loaves of Wonder bread, Skippy peanut butter and Welches grape jelly. She would make sandwiches for what seemed like forever, she would keep making sandwiches until everyone said they were full. The "bigs" could eat four sandwiches at a time. Lunch time was a daily production, but Muh always did it with a smile. It was our family time, those sandwiches would cancel the separation of the "bigs" and the "smalls" and allow us to just be one. After lunch, we would go back outside until our parents came to pick us up, group by group.

When I graduated to the first grade, my daily routine changed. Mom no longer worked as a teacher's aide and I was able to attend school with my older siblings so we all were transferred to St. Philip Neri Catholic School in Lynwood. Dad would get off his night job at 7:30 a.m., pick us up and drop us off to school. Jesse was in the eighth grade and Valencia in the sixth grade so they got to be on the same side of the campus. My first-grade class was closest to the back gate, across the yard from my brother and sister.

My mother would pick us up from school, while dad slept to get rest. I was back to being one of them on a daily basis, no more special time with mom. There were days when mom would tell us we could have a treat after school and we would all run to the back gate after school because we knew that meant a hamburger from McDonald's. The only thing is, we didn't have much money at the time, so instead of us each getting a hamburger, we would get one burger and have to split it four ways.

Mom would cut it as equally as she could but it seemed as though sometimes my piece was smaller, I guess because I was the smallest at the time. I thought,

"I can't wait until I am old enough to get my own burger, I am not sharing with anyone", or thoughts like, "If my brother and sister weren't here I would only have to share with my mom. I could have more."

I must have said that out loud one day because mom got upset and told me I was never satisfied and I was selfish. That hurt my feelings because I did not want to be selfish or ungrateful, I just wanted more burger. I felt ashamed for wanting more burger, I did not want to hurt my mother, especially since I watched her count pennies to make sure she had enough to buy the one burger. From that point on, I strived to act in such a way I would never be called selfish again.

My first-grade class was a fun class. On the first day of school, this boy name Travon told me I was pretty and I was his girlfriend. Travon was a cutie pie, he had a perfectly manicured afro that smelled like coconut oil, his clothes were always clean and pressed, he was smart, he could run fast and he could kick a ball farther than any other boy in the class. Out of all the girls in the class, he chose me. He was my introduction to noticing outer appearance does matter. I told my brother and sister, who were snitches so they told my parents. Instead of my parents saying I was too young for a boyfriend, they became friends with Travon's parents, and we began to hang out on a regular basis outside of school.

My friend at school in the first grade was Terrell, she was a cute and nice little girl. She liked Travon also but never seemed to mind when he would boldly announce I was his girlfriend. We worked together as a group and played together as a group. Travon and I didn't discuss at school the weekends we shared together while our parents sat up late playing cards and watching television at his house.

I guess Travon, even at a young age, wanted to be private, and I did not mention it because I did not want anyone to invade on our time. It was time I got to spend alone with him without classmates and it made me feel special the way I felt in kindergarten when I had mom to myself. After school, mom would drive us home and start preparing dinner. We were allowed to have a snack to hold us over until dinner was done. I loved to eat frozen bean and cheese Tina burritos. That was almost my daily after-school snack.

By the time I finished my snack, my brother and sister would be busy so I would go sit in the room alone and do homework, read a book or listen to the radio. During the school year, I didn't play outside much. I had enough time to do homework and chores. By the time I was done with that, it was time for dinner. My favorite meal for dinner was homemade beans or homemade smothered potatoes. I would eat until I literally felt as if I would explode! Mom cooked homemade meals daily.

Some days it seemed like she prepared some… what is it mixed with some I don't know, but it was always cooked with love and I ate it. My mother had a schedule to keep, so when it was dinner time, it was time to eat, hungry or not. I developed the habit of eating at "eating times" and not just when I was hungry.

Summertime was the most fun in Lynwood. My best friend's name was Elizabeth, we called her Mousey. She was funny and adventurous. She was the same age as I was but seemed so much more mature. Her parents would let her play outside as much as she wanted. She was a middle child, her older brother Anthony was close to my older siblings and her younger brother Lawrence was a year younger than us. She would come to my door early in the morning asking for me. Mom would always make me wait until the afternoon for some reason, so I would just be in the house listening to her have fun outside.

When I could go outside, I would go over to her and Lawrence, sometimes the boy across the street named Ramon would come over to play. We would roller skate, ride bikes, play kick ball, freeze tag, chase each other, put on talent shows and have a good time. The only break I had was when mom called me in for lunch. After lunch I would have to sit still for 30 minutes to let my food digest and then I was right back outside. Mousey got to eat outside. She would have Cup of Noodles all the time and she always made it look so delicious. My mom didn't buy Cup of Noodles, so I made myself a promise: When I could afford noodles, I would eat as many as I wanted.

Life Changes More

In second grade, my life changed even more. This was the year my parents had Demetria, my younger sister. Not only did I have to share mom and dad with the "bigs", now I had to share them with the first "small". Then, as if my dad was not at work enough, he took on yet another job, to make sure my mom could stay home to raise us and not have to leave the house. He worked to earn enough pay to keep a roof over our head, food in the house, clothes on everyone, utilities paid, and a car. That took two, sometimes three, jobs.

Dad was still working a lot during the week, so mom had to manage four kids and a household alone every day. On the weekends, everyone was drained, whether it was from going to school, maintaining a household or going to multiple jobs every day.
My father's way of relaxing was to go hang out with my uncles. My mom would always have him take me with him. The "bigs" were teenagers at this time so they were self-sufficient, which means she would only have to watch the baby, which after being with four kids all week was probably her way of relaxing.

Dad would drive to the liquor store for a six pack of beer and since I was the only child with him, I was able to get whatever I wanted. I always chose Cheetos, a plain Hershey bar and an Orange Crush soda. I would start eating as soon as we got back in the car. I could eat in peace and not have to share with anyone. My dad has never been a junk food eater.

We would go to abandoned train tracks on a street called Fernwood. He would park and began to wax his car. Sometimes my dad's brothers would come and they would bring the cousins my age. Contrary to the cousins on my mother side who I would be with at Muh's house, the cousins from my dad's side were real rebels.

Sherlinda grew up in Compton, so I always thought she was tough. Say something wrong to her she would cuss you out and threaten to have you beat up. Joseph and Toby were my uncle Terry's boys and he demanded his boys to be tough. Even if that meant street fighting every day, nobody was ever going to bully them or make them look less than a tough boy.

On these days I would hide my junk food in the car because if I had it out I knew they would take my snacks or they would punk me, telling me I thought I was better than them and out of guilt I would have to share with everyone. Either way, sharing would have been just like the McDonald's hamburger and the "bigs". I wanted something to call my own so I had to hide my stuff. As long as I had nothing we were on level playing fields. My cousins treated me as an equal. We would be over there for hours, I would walk the tracks because my older sister told me I could possibly find gold that fell off the train years ago.

I would listen to my dad and uncles speak to one another in their Creole language so the kids didn't have anything to run back and tell our mothers. I can still hear them laughing and teasing each other while I enjoyed the peacefulness of outside and my feeling of once again feeling like royalty because my dad was able to make me his only focus at that time, without him having to blur his vision by looking at my siblings.

On days when my cousins would be at the railroad with us and I had to hide my junk food, I would take the leftovers home. Of course when I walked in the house with Cheetos and a Hershey, the "bigs" would complain. Mom would get mad at dad because she didn't understand why he would buy me treats and none for my siblings. His logic was, they were not with him at the time. Although looking back, that was pretty messed up, but, it made me feel fulfilled.

My older siblings had one another, my younger sister had my mom, and I had my daddy and he treated me like a princess. Not my fault, my deal came with treats. Cheetos and Hershey became my favorite junk food, because I equate that with being special and an individual who was noticed and not just one of the kids. This pattern lasted for two years and then my parents had my little brother, Joaquin. Now I had two "smalls" to add to my two "bigs". I got even more lost in the mix. We had the bigs, we had the smalls and then there was me.

By this time, I was well conditioned to operate in a manner that became a subconscious habit and aided me in nurturing the fat genes, giving the strength to one day expand. Without any malice or ill intent, I was taught to eat whatever was in front of me when I was served. I was taught to eat when it was "eating time", not only when I was hungry. I was taught food, even junk food, can make me feel special.

The following two years, I decided to find outside activities to keep myself occupied. During my fourth through sixth grade years I joined Girl Scouts and played basketball and softball for the city of Lynwood. Unknowingly, being active helped me keep the Fat Genes intimidated and hidden inside of me.

Junior High School

Junior high school began in the seventh grade for me. This was a big change for me because my parents took me out of private school and sent me to a public school, Hosler Junior High in Lynwood. My parents were totally against the idea, but I begged and begged because the "bigs" attended public school and it just seemed like the cool thing to do. Little did I know, going to public school would open me up to a new world. Unlike Saint Philip Neri where I knew almost everyone because it was a small school and we all grew together, Hosler was filled with students from all over the city. Some were nice, others not so nice.

My family qualified for "free lunch" but if I was going to be popular and cool, I couldn't be seen in what the kids called the "county line", so I would save the allowance my father gave me to buy Laura Scudders cheese snacks, French fries and a fruit punch. That was my lunch for the first few weeks of school.

After the first few weeks I met other kids who also qualified for free lunch but did not want to be seen in the "county line". We figured out that if we wait until lunch was almost over, we could run into the cafeteria, get food and run out quickly because the line would have died down by then.

For the remainder of the seventh-grade school year and all throughout eighth grade, that is what we did. However, while my friends were walking around campus during the beginning of lunch, I was still in line to buy my Laura Scudders cheese snacks, French fries and fruit punch because when the bell rung at 12:10 p.m. my brain registered, "It is eating time, and you must eat!".

By 12:25 p.m. when my friends would meet me at the cafeteria, I really was not hungry but I still went in with them to get the free lunch, which most days included more French fries. I got my card stamped and received my tray of food. After a few bites, I was stuffed but I had to finish everything because "it was served to me on my plate".

My mother would pick me up from school every day, so outside of my modern dance class or P.E. class that lasted all of 20 minutes after roll call, I was not getting in any exercise. I was not aware of my Fat Genes at the time. I did not know how to be in tune with my body and listen to what it was telling me. Had I known then to be still and listens perhaps I would have heard the fat genes talking. I would have heard their conversation:

Introducing Fat Genes

FGs: "Alright Troops, now is the time for us to come together and figure out when would be a good time to introduce ourselves to the world through her. We laid dormant for the first 12 years of TT's life. We tried but we couldn't all jump out at once because that would have alarmed her parents and caused them to take drastic measures to get rid of us.

We got a little desperate when she was 9 years old, remember when she was alone with her father and we convinced her to borrow money from his pockets? He promised to take her to the store but he fell asleep. Our hope was built up so we used our evil powers to make her think since he was asleep, it would be OK to 'borrow' 50 cents from his pants pockets that were laying on the floor.

She snuck out and went to the convenience store for a peanut butter Twix. She quickly ate both sticks. We were satisfied but her conscience made her immediately feel like trash afterwards. She admitted she felt bad not because of the candy, that was delicious, she felt like trash because she stole, correction, "secretly borrowed" money from her dad to feed us. We tried to convince her that she was a kid and that is what kids do, but her Godly upbringing assured her that was not right. We learned on that day that we couldn't get her with feening, so we backed off to come up with a more slick way.

We thought 12 was a good age to come out at a slow and steady pace. Especially since she finally stopped playing softball and basketball for the city of Lynwood. All of that running, catching and throwing of the balls were quite intimidating, none of us wanted to be seen on her. Her exercise routine had completely stopped.

After a few laps during her P.E. hour at school, she stood around talking with friends for the remainder of class. We convinced her to eat Laura Scudders crunchy cheese snacks, French fries and fruit punches every day for lunch. Her mother picked her up from school and then she went home to sit to read or listen to the radio until it is time to eat. That was perfect and we made steady progress."

When I turned 14, I graduated to the ninth grade, which meant I transferred to high school. In the ninth grade was the first time I acknowledged the Fat Genes, but they were gentle and subtle. I paid attention to them because I wanted to wear the clothes all of the other kids were wearing but I could no longer fit the "affordable" clothes found at Zody's or Gemco, so I had to wear clothes that just fit over my hips, even if that meant pants that flood, bell bottoms (which are back in style now but in the 80's definitely were not in style), or pants in a size 20 but justified because they came from an Asian store and Asian clothes are smaller. No! Size 20 is a size 20 but the fat genes convinced me otherwise.

FGs: "We are looking good fellas, TT is fifteen years old now and weighs in at 190 pounds and she is only 5-feet-6 inches. A few people are beginning to take notice of us, did you hear what her brother-in-law asked her at dinner? Everyone was eating two or three tacos and he asked TT if she wanted TWELVE! He realized that we are here and we want her to feed us. We better slow down a bit, although his statement did not hurt her feelings, it did alarm her and she may begin to try to get rid of us. Let's take it easy for a while."

Chapter Two

The Plot of the Fat Genes

I was not happy with my weight, even at 190 pounds, but the Fat Genes convinced me I was fine. I allowed myself to ignore what the fat genes were whispering loud and clear to me. At the age of 15, my mother was still picking me up from school which eliminated my only form of exercise: walking home. My outer appearance was a sight to see. I had braces, my hair texture was thick and wooly, kids would call me a mix between the 80s singing group The Jets mixed with 80s singing group Five Star and the only way to keep my hair tamed without using a hot comb was to wear ponytails, but in the tenth grade, four pigtails with barrettes on the end were not cute.

My parents didn't want to hear my cries to let me change, I wanted to at least walk home from school so I could appear somewhat cool, but they insisted on keeping me on a tight leash. They wanted to keep me a baby. No one in school had time to tease me about my weight, they were too busy teasing me about the train tracks in my mouth and being too babied to walk home like a big kid.

I continued to eat and gain weight until one day out of the blue, my mother agreed with me and said I can walk home from school with my friends. I loved walking home, it gave me freedom. Little did I know that walking would jumpstart my first weight-loss journey. After my sophomore year in high school, my parents decided my summer would be spent living with my older sister and her family in Hampton, Virginia. This meant I did not have access to eat all of the junk food I wanted, no allowance from parents to buy snacks and no free rides anywhere.

In fact, I was uncomfortable eating in Virginia because I did not want my brother in-law to offer me twelve tacos again as if I were a human garbage disposal. Most days just to keep busy I would walk my nephew across the Air Force base to the playground and play with him until the sun went down. When I returned home to California months later, I had lost 55 pounds and sent the Fat Genes back into hiding.

I was not concerned with the fat genes because I seemed to have been able to control them and make them go away when I was tired of seeing them. Little did I know while they were in hiding there were still plotting and planning. They were scheming to come take over my world while I thought I was doing fine and living life. Now I wish I had been listening to them all along. Looking back, I can see how they had been planning a takeover all along. I could have prevented them from coming back with friends that were filled with the frustration of being forced to stay hidden for years!

Since birth, the Fat Genes were looking for a way to expose themselves to me. They started with my mind at a very early age by working with my family and influencing them to condition my mind to eat everything at the same time every day and to reward myself with junk food to make me feel loved and good. When I unintentionally fought them and won the battle of the bulge, they found strength and came back to me declaring a war.

When I started my junior year in high school, I was reminded of how the outer appearance can give a false feeling of control and sense of power. September 1988, I stepped on the school grounds of Lynwood High School a whole new person. I had my braces taken off over the summer, my sister straightened my hair before I left Virginia, and I had lost 60 pounds from walking and cutting back on my eating.

I became somewhat of a big deal on campus. Everyone wanted to know who the "new" fine girl was. I had to explain my unplanned weight loss story over and over. I had to convince others that it was really me they were speaking with. It was like I had a second chance to brand myself and I could be anyone I wanted. I had a lot of attention on me and it was all because I lost weight. It was vain, but I felt really good about myself, so much so, I could not hear the Fat Genes talking:

FGs: "I think we need to get back on the job now! Some of us have faded away. TT is sixteen now and her parents thought it would be a good idea to send her to stay with her sister in Hampton, Virginia so she could babysit her nephew while her sister worked at the local shoe store and her husband worked with the Air Force. What were they thinking? TT does not know a thing about babysitting. Every day she got her nephew dressed and they left the house walking to the play area on the Air Force base.

She would allow him to play on the slides, swings, and with balls for hours. Then they walked back home for lunch, which was normally a pitiful sandwich or soup and Teddy Grahams. After lunch they walked back to the playground and played until her sister returned home with dinner around 6 p.m. On most days she would have to carry her nephew back because he was wore out from all the playing. To top it off around 8 p.m. she goes to sleep! This is terrible, this is like exercising, this is like her playing sports again. Sixty of you are missing, we have to get you back!! We must invade her mind."

I was sitting alone one day reading a book when I heard a woman and man arguing. I stopped to listen and although I don't remember what they were arguing about, I do remember thinking it was silly. The woman kept talking and I remember thinking, why won't she shut up. I am not defending the man at all but I could tell she was saying all of the right things to push his buttons and I could feel the anger rising in him.

When I looked up, I remember seeing his arm drawn back with his hand in a fist position and he was aiming to knock her out. I don't know why I did this, but I jumped up and ran and got in the middle of them. The man told me to move and mind my own business and I yelled at him, "Well, stop fighting! I am trying to read!"

I don't know what came over me, I shocked myself when I heard the strength in my own voice. I don't know if that was God using me that day to be that woman's guardian angel or if I was just really into my book, but I do believe I may have saved that woman's life in that moment. That was my first taste of inner power and I loved it! Inner power is far better than power because of outer beauty.

By the time I was sixteen, I had fallen in love with control and power, except I did not know it. When someone mentioned the words control and power, I imagined a CEO of a Fortune 500 company, a wealthy person in a suit who had the ability to hire and fire people. That was not my role, so I did not associate the words with my personality. Yet, all along it was the fat genes convincing me my new vice did apply to me so that they could use my desire for control and power to benefit them further down the road. The FGs were adding ammunition for their troops while I was just existing, oblivious to the upcoming war.

At the start of my senior year in high school. I had the world at my fingertips. Most of the guys that I thought were cute or had hoped would talk to me in the ninth, tenth, and eleventh grades were now begging for my attention. I had school counselors pressuring me to sign up for city pageants, pretty girls wanting to be my friend. It was refreshing to feel so embraced and desired.

I was working at Kentucky Fried Chicken at the time and was tired of the smell and late hours. I applied for a job at Thrifty Drug Store but was told they were not hiring. When I went back to the store weeks later, I saw new faces. By this time, I was feeling myself, how dare they not hire me! I went looking for the manager, Mr. Knight. When I found him I asked, "What happened"? He gave some lame excuse, and I remember asking him to please consider hiring me when there is another opening.

Months later, I went into the store and saw more new faces! Once again, I looked for Mr. Knight and in so many words told him Thrifty's needed me to work for them. He literally told me to my face, I wanted to call you for the job but our district manager was here when you applied and he told me not to hire you because you were too pretty and would intimidate customers. I told him that was the silliest thing I had ever heard and if they wanted the store to stay open, they would hire me. In my mind, I was telling him I am a dependable and hard worker who would earn my paycheck honestly, but I think he took it as a threat because later that day he called and offered me a position as an ice cream clerk!

My looks had given me control over my life, I could demand what I wanted and get it. That was amazing! When I told Kentucky Fried Chicken I was quitting, they offered to pay for my schooling, to promote me to a lead, whatever I wanted but just don't leave. I had power.

When I was sixteen, my father bought me a 1980 orange Chevy Chevette. It came with an 8-track player but I was working so I took a full check to the Compton swap meet and paid them to install a Kenwood pullout radio. I was working, I had a car, I was on top of the world. One day while at work the district manager came in. I had not seen him and had no idea what he looked like. His name was Mr. Burke, he walked in and went straight into the storage room. I thought I was invincible so I followed him in the storage room and told him to leave, he did not belong there. He told me I should have called security but he appreciated me trying to protect the store.

We began to talk and I had the chance to tell him to never hinder someone's employment based on their looks alone. While he thought I would intimidate customers, it was quite the opposite, people came into the store because we had an awesome crew. Everyone was always helpful and friendly.

Having good looking employees was a bonus that drew in customers. He apologized and thanked me for being one of the hardest workers in the company. It felt so good to feel equipped with power and control. So I thought, in reality, my parents still had the power. I was still living with them and they were still treating me like a baby.

As a high school senior, I was not allowed to speak to boys on the house phone, in fact I could hardly speak to females friends on the phone because my parents felt if I was with these friends all day at school and work, what could we possibly have to talk about on the phone? I was not allowed to go out on weekends or days off to just hang out, that was unheard of.

If I was invited to an outing or over to someone's house, there had to be a woman in the house. If a friend was being raised by a single father, I did not bother asking. My mother would have to meet their mother first, interrogate her and wait a few days for a decision. It took away my control and power. I hated it! I was being called "homie", "square" and worst of all, guys were calling me conceited because I wasn't giving out my number.

My power from outer appearance was fading away, the very people that had flocked to me were now turning away from me because I "was too good" to accept invitations from them. I had to find a way to get control back.

Cedric

I was allowed to attend my senior prom with a guy from my government class named Cedric.

Although we had attended the same school since our freshman year, I had never seen him before. He was tall, dark and had the best smile with big, white, perfect teeth. One day we were in class and people were talking about senior pictures and the upcoming prom. I didn't say anything, I just listened because I was not sure if my parents would allow me to attend.

After school, I was walking home with my friend Krystal and her friend Karen. I was telling Krystal all about this guy in my class that I had never seen before but how I wanted him to ask me to the prom. I figured he would never ask me but it didn't hurt to fantasize about it.

The next day in class, Cedric came to me and told me his sister Karen had informed him of all the gushing I was doing the day before while walking home with her and our friend Krystal. I wanted to faint! He thought it was cute and asked me to the prom. I knew for sure my parents would have said no, but surprisingly they did not.

Cedric and I started planning for the prom and eventually started saying we were a couple around campus. I say around campus because off campus, I was not allowed to date, so weekend movies were out. I went to his house to study a few times, but my mom was always lurking and demanding I come right back home.

Cedric felt my frustrations of not having any control or power over my freedom and said he would join the military and send for me to get away. Seemed like a perfect plan to me. I knew I wanted my control and power back so I was willing to do whatever it took. As soon as we graduated high school Cedric enlisted in the Army.

A war started, Desert Storm. He was sent to Saudi Arabia and I was left home. I was focused on school and work. Most days I daydreamed of how to gain my control and freedom back, since I learned my outer appearance wasn't the true key to obtaining it.

I waited two years for Cedric to come back and when he appeared he came back stronger and more mature. He asked for my hand in marriage. I said yes and my parents lost it! How could I agree to marry someone I only went to the prom with? I didn't care, I knew I liked Cedric, I enjoyed reading the letters we wrote, he was smart, he was funny, and he was a man of his word.

He said he was coming to get me and he came back. We were engaged and he asked to send for me in a few months. The problem was, we were not married and my parents would never allow for me to fly to another state to visit a man, so I declined. Shortly after our letters started to slow down, my work schedule picked up so I could not be home to speak to him on the phone (no cell phones at this time).

About a year later, I learned Cedric married another girl named Tonya that he met in the Army. I was crushed. I was still wearing my engagement ring and had been working and going to school, counting down the days for us to get married and for me to regain my control and freedom and in a blink of an eye that dream vanished.

I continued to work and go to school but the feeling of me never gaining control and power back was nagging at me daily. The Fat Genes are pretty clever, they were not luring me to food at this time but they were conditioning my brain to believe I had to have control and power. I attempted to date other men but my parents always shut me down.

Oddly, my older two siblings never experienced this type of "shelter". Both of my older siblings were allowed to date freely and both were congratulated when they married young and started families. I, on the other hand, was the chosen one. Work and school were the only freedom I was allowed, but even that was on a schedule. I could not leave too early for school and definitely had to return home immediately after work. Most days my schedule was school 7 a.m. to 12 p.m. and work 1:30 p.m. to 10 p.m. Even at the age of 20 my curfew was 10 p.m., so after-work hangouts were never allowed.

I was still fighting to figure out a way to gain my freedom. The thought of going away to college came to mind, but who was going to pay for it? Joining the military was not appealing. The only two females I would have lived with were not looking for roommates. I felt like I would be trapped and sheltered forever. Powerless and absolutely no control.

Fighting for Freedom

Carlos came into my job, Thrifty Drug Store. He had just returned from serving his time in the United States Air Force and looked really handsome. We attended high school together but never really talked. We would speak at school because our siblings were married to one another, but he never showed any interest in getting to know me, so I paid him no mind. He was sort of popular on campus. He was a football player, a great dancer and somewhat of a loud mouth, a character for sure.

He always had a girlfriend and was always running around. The military does something to young men because like Cedric, he came back more mature and wise. Surprisingly, when Carlos was in the store he asked me out on a date. I accepted, believing my parents would approve because my sister was married to his brother and they came from a good family.

The next day, I asked my parents. It was an instant no. They didn't see him as my sister's brother-in-law, they saw him as a man. They had to use their control and power over me, so they shut that down real fast. I cried and begged to go out. Eventually, I was allowed to go out with Carlos. We went to a Dodger game and I had a blast! The next week, Carlos asked if I wanted to go to a game again. Of course, baseball is one of my favorites. Once again, it was a struggle at home, parents gave me hell about asking to go out. I went and again had a good time, but then Carlos wanted to go out to eat after the game. I knew this was not a good idea because the agreement with my parents was I would go to the ballgame and come straight home.

I knew my mother who does not like baseball would be watching the game just so she could see what time it ended and then time my drive from Los Angeles back to Lynwood. I was too embarrassed to tell Carlos about my lack of power and control so I took my chances and went to eat. We went to a quick diner, Ruby's, ate a burger and got home. My mom was waiting at the door. I was forbidden to see Carlos ever again.

I was twenty years old and felt as if I had no control over my life. The desire to feel like I had control and power was killing me, I had to think quick and do something. Carlos invited me to move in with him and I told him I wanted my independence but not get killed for it. My father would have broken both of our necks if I would have "shacked up". So, I told Carlos, the only way I would move in with him is if he married me. We were married two weeks later. I ran away. I wanted my power and I knew I had Carlos' support because he agreed to go along with this crazy plan. Me saying yes and meaning it equated power with being a daredevil and that was what he was attracted to.

I grabbed a prom dress off the Cerritos mall clearance rack, he grabbed a suit from Sears, we called our best friends Myra Fields and Aric Bundage to be a witness and we were married August 16, 1992. Literally, two weeks after the proposal. The beginning of my marriage was wonderful. We didn't really operate as husband and wife but more like young, free kids. We moved to Chino, California and I was able to go and come as I pleased. We went to late night movies, talked until early morning, we would go to the gym late at night, we had fun!

I felt in control and that was I wanted. I thought I had gained ultimate power. But I was frustrating my FGs and fueling my addiction for control and power that would later benefit the FGs. I weighed 132 pounds and I was happy! For my twenty-first birthday we went to Hawaii and that is when the FG's ran out of patience with not being seen. They started back up with their meetings and conversations:

FGs: "Well, it has been five years and we are still in hiding! Our assignment was to take over TT's body and kill her! What are we waiting for? She is twenty one years old now and smaller than she has ever been! Over half of you wimps have left her body and are nowhere to be found. She married this man that goes with her to the gym every day and she is walking on lunch breaks at work. I told you guys we must invade her mind because her physical activity has been on point for the past several years. It is time we allow her to see her real world and get her out of this perfect life fantasy she thinks she is living. It is our turn to shine!"

Chapter Three

Losing Control

Life had a funny way of pulling out my strengths and teaching me about my power. I got married when I was twenty years old. I chose to marry because I felt my parents were entirely too strict with me and I hated feeling powerless. My older siblings were married and had moved away by this time. At home were just the "smalls" and me. Dad was still always working and mom was busy with the "smalls". Yet my parents still managed to find time to control my freedom of expression. Regardless of how badly I wanted my power, I did not want to disappoint my parents or shame my family name, so I married because it was the Christian thing to do. I was fighting for a power, yet leaving them with control to dictate the conditions I leave under.

Marriage or be disowned. It is ironic now looking back. The FGs were steadily loading ammunition and I had no clue. The joy of being married quickly ended. He, like me, was under the spell of wanting power and control but having parents or in his case a parent hold it in her hands. I was operating as a free spirit and he was still operating under his mother's demands. I just gained my control and power and being with someone who did not have the same was a major turn-off.

I respected him for loving his mother but resented him for always catering to her and treating me like a second thought. I never got the chance to live as his wife. He moved his mother in shortly after we were married and he went back to being the little boy I knew in high school.

His every move had to be approved by her. He was still a nice guy, but simply not man enough for me. Instead of him having FGs to drive him, he had uncontrollable lust for other women. So on top of competing with his mother, I had to compete with ex-girlfriends, new girlfriends, his coworkers and neighbors. This left me with the feeling of overwhelming stress. I felt stuck in a bootleg marriage because I did not believe in divorce and I was unknowingly welcoming FGs take over.

Carlos and I managed to stay married for about a year and six months before we realized we were better off as friends, because of my rushed decision and my parents controlling my freedom, I didn't learn who he was until we were married. We decided to divorce on friendly terms and all would have been well, except for the fact that shortly after we returned from Hawaii, I learned I was pregnant with his child. He decided he wasn't ready to be a father because he had not finished chasing after girls and had yet to discover his freedom from his mother.

When we were legally divorced he thought that meant he got to leave me and our unborn baby. I had gotten pregnant around my 21st birthday on a trip to Hawaii. The FGs figured they could disguise their attack through a pregnancy. I was aware of them this time. I was aware and knew to listen to them communicate. I would communicate back with them in my head.

The Genes at Work

FGs: Talking to one another, "Great news! We overheard TT tell her husband she is pregnant! Now is our time. We can get in her head and make her think it is OK to eat whatever she wants because it is not for her, it is for the baby!! Yes, this is a perfect plan!!

"It is working guys, she is not even 3 months along and she is back to her pig-out eating habits. She eats a big breakfast at home, then on her ten-minute break at Thrifty's she goes next door to Pioneer Chicken for a snack, Wienerschnitzel for lunch, eats a large bag of Raisinets while she is working, and then goes home to eat dinner, a big dinner! "That is over 4,000 calories a day. This is amazing!! By her 9th month we will all be back, she will think it is the baby and we will stay with her forever, or at least until we kill her off. Finally, we can complete our mission."

TT: Hello, FGs! I recognize you this time. The doctor told me today that I must get rid of some of you. He said you will harm my baby and give me diabetes. I don't believe the doctor and his scary description of you, so, here is the deal, I have to keep my baby happy. If she craves it, I'll eat it. After all, I am supposed to gain weight while pregnant, but while I am giving birth, I will need all of you extra FGs to come out as well. So what if I have gained one hundred pounds with this pregnancy.

FGs: "Did you guys hear that? We knew she would do anything for her unborn child. We got her mind fellas. This was too easy! I see there are 100 of us in here, good thing she is pregnant and her skin stretched, otherwise we would be crowded in her body. If she thinks she is kicking us out, she is in for a rude surprise!"

Happiest Day of My Life

August 24, 1993, the happiest day of my life! I gave birth to the most beautiful little girl my eyes have ever beheld. On this day, I saw love in the flesh. Her name is Charity Lanette. She was absolutely worth the 100-pound gain, but now that she is here, it is time to get rid of them.

FGs: "Did you guys hear that? She will get rid of us. We must do something, we are comfortable in her body now. I bet she will start going to the gym like she used to with her husband again. We cannot have that!! Let's do something."

The thought of being a single mother was taking its toll on me. I was young and afraid. The FGs thought it would be a perfect time to start to win the war. So they picked up mission "control her brain" into overtime. They found sneaky ways to throw hurdles in front of me that they thought would play a part in me losing the war with them.

FGs: "OK, that was a bit drastic, a cheating husband that wants to run out on his wife and child! FGs, that was harsh but it is understandable we have been being careful for almost 22 years now and if sending her into a depression to make her overeat and keep us is what it took for her to be ready to accept us, then so be it."

TT: I am OK with my husband leaving, as long as I have my baby. I will work hard and shower her with so much love, and we will be just fine. My focus is on providing the best life possible for her. By the time my daughter, Charity, was a month-old Carlos had managed to move most of his stuff out and create a schedule that would not require him to come home much. I went back to work when Charity was only six weeks old, which scared me something terrible. She was an infant who could not speak and I had to leave her with a babysitter I did not know.

I moved to Chino and my parents still lived in Lynwood. That is approximately 40 miles apart so I could not ask my parents to watch my daughter. I asked the mail carrier who delivered mail to the Thrifty's I was working at who watched her daughter while she worked and she gave me the number to Ms. Helen, a lady who ran a daycare out of her house.

I was a nervous wreck for the first six months of going back to work. At this time, I was working in Ontario, CA. and my hours were 10:30 a.m. to 7 p.m. I was so consumed with worry of my baby and if she was OK, most days I would forget to feed myself. I went from being a sheltered independent child to being a divorced single mom in a matter of two years and all before I was twenty-three years old. Things happened so fast I did not have time to dwell on a divorce, the women my ex cheated on me with, his mother who acted like she was one of the women he was cheating with, Carlos tricking me into signing away my rights to our home in Chino, where my next meal was coming from, how was I doing, who was going to care about me?

I had no time to address those things, my one and only focus was on my daughter. Loving her was easy, I fell in love with her the day the nurse practitioner told me I was a few weeks pregnant. What I didn't know was how was I going to muster up enough strength and wisdom to care for her mentally, physically, financially? Days turned into weeks, weeks into months, months into years and God provided a way each step. I discovered a strength in me I never knew I had.

My job paid enough to cover rent, utilities and gas to put in the car to get to work, but I had to teach myself how to get food and clothes. I remembered at my prenatal appointments they always had a storage room filled with samples of full-size cans of Enfamil (expensive baby formula). After Charity was born, I would still go to the hospital and ask for two cans of Enfamil so my baby could try. I would then take the samples to the grocery store, tell them my baby only drinks Carnation Good Start and they would allow me to exchange one can of Enfamil for two cans of Carnation Good Start.

I taught myself if there is an open bag of diapers on the shelf, the store manager at Thrifty's would permit me to purchase the $13 bag for $5. I found the clearance racks at TJ Maxx for clothes before TJ Maxx became a popular store. I was on a mission to never allow my child to miss a beat and we survived. I learned to survive on Tuna Helper. A one-dollar box would be my breakfast and dinner every day. I would often skip lunch.

I called Carlos a few times to ask for help but by the time he would come around it was too late. I would tell him on Monday, our daughter would need something by Friday and he would come by on Sunday. What was the point? Eventually, he stopped coming because he said every time he showed up, I had the situation under control. This would irritate me to no end. I don't think he still gets it today. If I say a child needs milk by Friday, and he shows up on

Sunday, was she supposed to starve all day Saturday? Of course I would have figured it out in his absence, any good mother would have.

This was another tactic, the FGs used for control of my thought process. I am not one to procrastinate, if work needs to be done, I will do it right away. By any means necessary. This was OK for my daughter, but the perception of "Tonya can handle it" spilled over in my adult personal life and work life. It was another tactic of the FGs.

FGs: "Guys, I think we messed up! We did not factor in the focus TT can have when she really wants something. She said she will work hard, that means she will get 2 sometimes 3 jobs to support her daughter, she won't have time for us! OK, we can use that to our advantage later on, we can convince her she is overworked and too tired to cook or eat healthy, that is an easy fix. What we forgot about was the fact that she does not know how to babysit!!! She has been so focused on feeding her daughter baby food, she is forgetting to feed us! She wakes up early to feed the baby, she walks all day standing on her feet then she rushes to the sitter to get her daughter, just to go home and cater to her until they fall asleep. The good news is she forgot about exercising and her focus is not on herself, so if we could just get her to eat, she won't notice and we will be fine. The bad news is, she has not figured out how to feed the child and eat, she is starving us. Most of you have left us again. Our plan might backfire! Let's gather together and think of another plan."

By the time Charity was a year old, I had lost 90 of the 100 pounds. I was aware of the extra FGs and I knew I did not want them there. I never set out to lose them on purpose, I was lost in my new world of being a mother and I did not even notice when they started going back into hiding. I got rid of them without trying. My daughter and I were still living in Chino at the time, in the townhouse Carlos and I sought out to purchase together years prior. In the divorce, the judge ordered I keep the house because I was going to have sole custody of Charity.

We stayed there for a couple of years before the mortgage hit the larger part of the adjustable mortgage rate. Being young and a single mother, I panicked. Carlos convinced me to "give" the house back to him by doing what the courts call a "nunc pro tunc" ruling. He took over the house payments and moved in with his new wife and her daughter, never once showing a sign of caring about where his daughter and I would now live. I was angry, hurt and relieved at the same time. I felt like a failure but was happy I did not have to figure out how to pay for a higher mortgage, car note, car insurance, day care and care for a child all at the same time, by myself! The FGs put this in their storage room of power over me for later use.

Time to Move

Charity and I moved to an apartment in Buena Park. She was able to talk at this point so I was comfortable in placing her in a new daycare and I stayed focused on making our life work! At this time I was working for Thrifty's but in Long Beach. I was not given a set work schedule so I placed her in a daycare near my parents so I had someone to pick her up in case I was scheduled to work later than 6 p.m., the closing time of the daycare.

The days I got off work at 7 p.m., my mother would pick my baby up for me. By the time I got to Charity, my mother would have already fed her dinner with my siblings, the "littles". I would be so exhausted from work, I almost always opted out of eating a home-cooked meal prepared by mother, I just wanted to grab Charity, her diaper bag and get home.

My dinner became a quick meal from a local fast food place. It got so bad that when the owners of the local burger stand, Bob's Burger, would see me, they would start preparing my order. I felt like a celebrity. While others waited in line to place an order, I just walked up, paid and got my food. This was before eateries had call ahead ordering. I felt like I had power. The older Charity got, the more money we needed.

While I was with Thrifty's Drug Store I was blessed to be put through a Pharmacy Technician program where I became licensed by the state of California. I needed more money to survive so after nine years, I left the job that required me to stand up all day and move around for a desk job at Prescription Solutions in Costa Mesa, CA. This was a great advantage for the FGs.

Charity and I then moved into a condo-style apartment in Anaheim. My next-door neighbor was my best friend Myra. We had a blast having one another next door. In the beginning we were like Lucy and Ethel running next door for great laughs. It became a routine for us to make late night runs to Denny's for brownie ala modes.

As the years passed, our lives became more demanding with work and children. Although we lived next door to one another, I rarely saw Myra. We would have to schedule time to hang out and that was always surrounded by food. We always went out to eat, that was our escape. After a few years, Myra moved away, but I carried on our tradition of Denny's dashes and going out to eat for relaxation.

As I grew older, I gained more survival wisdom and strength. If Charity wanted or needed something out of my budget, I found a way to earn more money. In addition to my day job, I was a licensed notary, I would buy name brand (knock-off) purses at wholesale prices and sell them from my desk, I would buy one music cd and exchange it for five bootleg CDs of other artists from this girl that lived in my apartment building and then I would sell the bootleg CDs for $5 each to people in my office (I apologize now to all my music artist friends that I now have in my life). I was unstoppable. Give me a problem and I solved it.

Just like with Carlos and his failure to show up for our daughter, I figured things out and was succeeding. Today, I am grateful to Carlos for leaving us alone because it forced me to learn how to think fast on my feet and it gave me the opportunity to unintentionally and subconsciously show Charity how to survive. One time, Charity had an assignment due which required it to be typed. We could not afford a computer so I would put her name on the list to reserve a computer at the library.

Unfortunately, so did a lot of other parents, so her reservation time would be fifteen minutes before closing time. I was just getting off work, it was just not a good plan, so being the problem solver, I am, we bought a typewriter. She had no idea what it was but I taught her and our problem was solved. When Charity needed doll clothes, we cut up our old clothes and I taught her how to create a pattern and hand sew an outfit together. When extra bills were due or she needed money for activities at school, I found a hustle, earned extra money and the problem was solved. I was too busy "making it" to focus on me.

My work life was blossoming. After a few years at the Prescription Solutions Pharmacy Helpdesk, I learned about medical claims and transferred to the claims department to become a claim processor. This is where my "Don't procrastinate, get it done attitude" came into play. This is a blessing and a curse. While my coworkers sat around discussing the latest edition of the Steve Harvey radio show, I would be working. My claims would always be done on time, quota met and accuracy level high. Instead of getting more money, I got more work. The company figured since I was so good at my job, I could handle more responsibility while others got to slack off. I did not say anything, instead I internalized my frustrations adding fuel to the FGs weaponry. I began snacking at my desk.

In a few years I was promoted and became an auditor and I made it look like I had everything under control. What I know now is people will use you up until you say stop. I was working like a slave and stressing and gaining weight for a company that kicked me right out the door when they learned my work could be done cheaper in Ireland. Friends would call me with problems. I solved them. Especially men problems. I was the only one in my circle who had been married and divorced. Single mother problems? I had an answer because I felt I had been through it all. Job problems? I could talk to some people and get them hired. There was nothing I couldn't do. I had strength plus power and I was unstoppable. Looking from the outside, I was in total control of my life. I taught myself to bargain shop and used my hustle money to travel with my daughter and shop. I spent the remainder of my 20's working on being the "perfect mom" and "best worker." I never focused on me.

Unknowingly, I was successfully allowing the FGs to take over my brain and give me a false belief that I had everything under control. The truth was, I was surviving. My mother instilled so much faith and wisdom in five children, she taught us how to keep a house warm, how to create a meal, how to entertain without a dime. My father taught us how to be dedicated to work, how to be responsible, and how to sacrifice self so that someone else would be fine. I was living on autopilot based on the lessons learned in my youth while the FGs were training me how to mentally sabotage my future.

By the time I was thirty, I had mentally worn myself out. I had convinced myself that I was doing everything alone and I was over it. I was tired and I wanted physical help. In addition to being a single mother and a dedicated worker for a corporate company, I was a sister friend to several people, an usher at church, a cheer mom, a student, and was seeking to run my own business. Still, I never took time for myself and I was steadily gaining weight. I was too exhausted mentally to think about exercising, and if I did want to exercise, when was I going to?

I was up at 5:30 a.m., as soon as my feet hit the floor I was rushing to get dressed for work, get Charity dressed for school, comb hair, prepare her lunchbox, drop her off to before-school care, and rush to clock in for work. After work, it was pick her up or go to Compton College for a night course, go home, homework, chores, etc. By 10 p.m., I was sleepy. There were brief moments when my higher self would try to force me to pay attention to myself, but the FGs always had a clever comeback. They came with what seemed to be perfect solutions. I never took the time to really listen and pay attention to what the FGs were doing.

For example, working in corporate America, you have to dress a certain way, so when my clothes began to get too tight and I decided I would exercise and change my eating habits, the FGs would rally together and come up with a plan. Had I been paying attention, I would have heard them say:

FGs: "First, let's get in her head and convince her she is fine just the way she is, this way she will not continue think of those of us who have managed to come back to live in her body. We can start by telling her she should treat herself to something nice since she works so hard. Let's send her to the mall to buy a few outfits! She loves fitted suits so we have to convince her the brand suits she wants are not in her budget right now, then we will email her coupons to a store that sells pretty clothes that come only in stretchy materials, this way, she can love the way she looks and more of us can creep back on her without her noticing because she will continue to be able to fit the clothes. Brilliant!"

TT: I was thinking to myself, "I really need new clothes for work". Miraculously, I would check my emails and there would be coupons. NY&Co, spend $300 on clothes, save $175! Without taking a moment to recognize it was a part of a bigger plan, I would head to the mall that day and shop. I was convinced I was doing right by me and being responsible because I would leave with really cute clothes and I was getting four outfits for the price of one.

FGs: "It is working guys, she just bought four pair of pants that will still fit comfortably even after we get 60 of our lost fat genes back. Oh, and let the guys know if they want to bring 10 or 15 of their friends with them when they come back, they are welcomed to because we have accomplished our mission to overpower her mind and she is totally ignoring what is happening to her." By this time, I was 32 and weighed 180 pounds.

Chapter Four

May I Take Your Order?

Somewhere along my life journey I adapted to a self-sabotaging servant mentality. I became so engulfed with making sure everyone around me was fine, I often forgot about me. I was neglecting myself for the sake of other people's desires and dreams. I guess this could stem from being a middle child. I was accustomed to just being there while quietly doing whatever it takes to keep everyone happy. It became normal for me not to ask for what I wanted, because nothing was ever "supposed" to be about just me.

Growing up, if I did ask for something specifically for me, I was called selfish. The one title I hated the most. That was probably the most hurtful thing I have ever been called. Me, selfish? Impossible! I know my heart and all of my intentions and I cannot recall one time when I set out to be purely selfish, yet still I trained myself not to ask for much or ask for anything at all.

In retrospect, I can see me asking for something specifically was added pressure on my parents who were already struggling to maintain the household.

My father worked hard to provide what his family needed and worked even harder to ensure we got what we wanted during Christmas time and our birthdays. Rather than being told no when I asked for something throughout the year or outside of "normal" special days, I was called selfish. No harm was intended but I did not know how to process that.

I mentally instructed myself to never request anything or act in a manner that would portray me as selfish. I carried that into my adult life and my enemy FGs added my belief to their private storage of weapons of mass destruction. I was also raised to be humble. It is shameful and sinful to have pride. What I did not know is there is a difference between being prideful and being proud of myself. Another tactical device for the FGs to sabotage me. There are certain behaviors a person can demonstrate that will literally embarrass me. These people have absolutely nothing to do with me, yet I am embarrassed.

I remember watching an episode of I Love Lucy and hiding behind my pillow because I was so ashamed of Lucy. That seems silly, but it is the way I am wired. Well, in real life, when people did something I felt was embarrassing or I did not agree with, I would shy away. I did not want to be seen with such actions. When it was a family member that displayed such an action, I was told I could have been the star in the movie "Imitation of Life". Again, life-changing, hurtful words!

I was never ashamed of my family, especially my immediate family, but if they were talking loud in public, popping gum in public, etc., these behaviors did not fit me so I walked away. After it was embedded in my head that I was "acting funny", I again learned to adapt and accept behavior from others that I did not want to approve of. I never wanted anyone to feel as if I thought I was "too good" to be around them. That became another weapon that I supplied for the FGs to be used against me in my adult life.

By nature, I am a giver, a problem solver and solutions oriented. So I would often attract people who are takers. I allowed people into my life who took and took until I became completely empty. The FGs are just like Satan, they are the author of confusion and they had me totally confused. I was living and giving to others and allowing them to gather and plan my destruction. They kept me in the dark about myself and had me constantly eating junk in an effort to fill a bottomless pit of empty emotions.

I could not acknowledge my emotions because that meant I would have had to focus on me, that would be selfish and the FGs knew I would think that. I did not make wise choices about the people I allowed in my circle because that meant I would be acting as if I was "too good" to be around some individuals. Instead, I welcomed everyone and ate away any pain or grief they may have caused me.

This mentality carried over into my dating life. I have heard many women state, after a divorce they felt "not good enough so they couldn't be loved". That was never my intentional thoughts, I knew I deserved to be loved, the FGs picked up on me being emotionally unfit and used my brainwashed mindset to attract less-than-worthy suitors to love me, all so they could continue to chip away at my health. Dating was never an issue for me. Dating the right man was the issue.

A few years after my divorce, I dated a bank teller. He was a nice guy but had no drive or determination in life. His ultimate goal in life was to outlive his parents so he can become owner of their home. Watching him live was draining to me, I could not grasp his concept of survival. I was a single mother, drove a newer car, had my own apartment, paid bills on time, paid daycare, was a part-time college student and still had spare money.

Meanwhile, he lived with his parents, had never been married, no children, had an old car that sometimes started, wore the same clothes almost daily and never had any money because he said he was paying his way through school and had two more classes than me. My FGs convinced me I was not above his way of thinking and I should hang in there with him. It was not until he offended my FGs that he got the boot.

Fat Genes Speak Out

One day, he asked me out to lunch. Well, I was already preparing to cook chicken breast and mushroom soup at home. I told him and he said no don't cook that, I am on my way over so we can eat together. I thought he was going to arrive with food, instead he arrived empty-handed and said he wanted me to wait so we could cook together. I was irritated but I hid my emotions because I had trained myself to accommodate those around me and put my wants and feelings on the back burner. I seasoned the chicken, just the way I like it but behind my back he added a ton more black pepper.

Then, when I asked him to open the can of soup, he literally spit on the can. His excuse was the can may have been dusty and he wanted to "spit shine" it. This triggered the FGs because they knew I was not going to eat anything that someone spit on. This was worse than seeing my cousins' chewed up food at my grandmother's table. I allowed him to stay, he ate and I trashed the rest of the food. I found pleasure in watching him hold his throat while he ate the extra spicy chicken he destroyed. This was on a Saturday, by the time Monday came, the FGs had convinced me we did not need him messing up our meals and he could no longer be a part of our lives. Monday morning, I walked into his bank and told him thank you for the past year but I did not want to see him anymore.

I should have recognized the power of the FGs then, but I was blinded. This guy stole my daughter's PlayStation, never had any money, drove a car that allowed me to see the street through the floor when we drove, lived with his parents waiting on their death, and I tolerated it all because I did not want to offend him, but when he offended the FGs I was subconsciously advised to let him go. The FGs made me feel as if they were my true friends. After dating the banker, they really began to comfort me. I wish I had heard them whispering to one another:

FGs: "That is it that is really it. We have lost so much time. Thirty-two years, count them, thirty-two and we have not sustained one accomplishment! We add ourselves to her then we go back into hiding, come out and back into hiding. We need a plan once and for all that will take TT out for good!"

Over the years, the FGs and I grew together, we adjusted to our coexistence and fulfilled one another's needs. The foundation to destroy me had already been built by the FGs, but it was at this time that they activated and really began to work. I developed "Shallow Hal" eyes, I looked in the mirror and no matter what weight I was I only saw the 135-pound version of myself. I allowed them to trick me into believing we were in a loving relationship.

My Fat Genes work well together and they each know how to let one another take lead on any given day. Some days the Fat Gene that only wants chips all day is the boss, other days the Fat Gene that wants

Hershey candies is in charge, there are a few that demand Taco Bell, WingStop, and other fast food several times a week, and I know there is a committee of Fat Genes that thrives on Rock Star fruit punch energy drinks.

Those are the strongest ones, even when I am not tired they convince me to drink a Rock Star. I literally felt the immediate gratification when I digested those high calorie drinks. They work so well together and were so smooth and slick with their arrivals, I did not notice them, in fact it seems as if 60 of them outwardly appeared overnight. The FGs got real insistent and comfortable. They even tried to make me comfortable with allowing them to hold a permanent residence in my mind and on my body.

I'll admit, in the beginning it was a fairytale connection, both parties were so willing to give each other what they wanted and both parties never ended a day feeling unfulfilled. The Fat Genes merely wanted to be fed an abundance of junk food, while I simply wanted to feel loved, comforted, and in control.

As the years passed, I gladly gratified them with every fast food joint imaginable, chips, cookies, candy, sodas, and fruit juices. The Fat Genes were more than happy to leave me feeling soft, warm, cuddly, and loved. Life was great, so I thought. My Fat Genes were ready for the take down. Now that I was at 240 pounds, dating was certainly the very last thing on my mind. I was content with raising Charity alone, getting her through school, going to school for my degree, working as a medical claims auditor, running side businesses and eating snacks.

Then one day while shopping, I ran into a guy from high school. He was cute, drove a nice vehicle, had a decent job as a computer repairman, appeared to love his children and still called me beautiful even though I weighed 240 pounds. We talked for a short while, he interacted nicely with Charity so it was a no-brainer to say yes when he asked me out on a date.

He remembered where my parents lived from seeing me walk home in high school. I mentioned to him that I was going to stop by to see my parents later that day, and by the time I got there he had left me a gift. It was a bottle of Wings perfume and a note saying it was great seeing me and he couldn't wait to see me again. I was on cloud nine. Not even while I was married had anyone bought me a gift, just because. It felt good.

The FGs are slick, I already knew but I was not hip to their game. They came in at a different angle with this one. They were not going to attract anyone who was going to destroy our eating arrangements and they knew bringing someone without drive or goals would remind me of the banker and I would not give it a chance, so they came at a completely different angle with an end-game plan that would take me out for sure with him.

I was in no way prepared for the destruction I was opening myself up to with him. As usual, the FGs were trying to be patient so they decided to allow computer guy and I to build a relationship before they would drop the bomb on me. Computer guy was smart, funny, adventurous and loved to eat out at fancy places. I grew up in California but he took me to restaurants I had never heard of. He was a romantic and he loved junk food. It was a perfect match for all three of us, him, me, and my FGs.

If I was looking through a magazine and saw something I liked, all I had to do was mention it and I would have it. He bought me my first Coach bag, all because I said it was cute. He would bring me clothes because he thought they would look nice on me. He bought my daughter bikes, toys, clothes, whatever he bought his children, he bought for my daughter. He took off work to attend my daughter school functions with me. He attended church, he prayed, dressed well, always smelled good and had great teeth. He was perfect on the surface.

Behind closed doors I saw all sorts of red flags to run, but the FGs convinced me to stay. If I said I was going to the nail shop, he would demand that I wait for him to pick me up and take me because he wanted to pay AND he wanted to be sure I was really going to the nail shop. After our trips to the nail shop we almost always went to eat at Versailles, a restaurant that serves my favorite Cuban food. While I hated that I would have to wait for him, the FGs knew that we would eat a great meal afterwards so they reminded me of my battle not to be "selfish" and to always consider others.

If I was at his house, he would always cook a meal, mostly deep-fried stuff. He would prepare my plate without asking if I was hungry, and even if I was not hungry, I would eat with him because he thought it was rude if I did not and the FGs reminded me that it was my moral obligation to eat at eating time and to finish everything placed in front of me. I could only go out with him, or if I went out I had to have one of our children with me, or I could only go a short distance with one of my female friends that he approved of and I had to be near a pay phone to answer his pages whenever he beeped me on my pager.

He would go as far as to leave his job in the middle of the day so he could drive 20 miles to my job to have lunch with me, just to make sure I was not eating with a male co-worker. At his house, I had to use the restroom in his bedroom with the bathroom door open to make sure I was not writing a letter (we did not have cell phones) to another man. The biggest red flag was when I would catch him having full-on conversations with his deceased uncle. This dude was nuts but the FGs made me stay loyal by reminding me that I could not think I was better than him and leave, I could not be selfish and desert his children who had come to love me, nor interrupt the relationship he had built with my daughter.

This crazy man even broke into my home one day. I had gone roller blading with my best friend Myra and he was paging me like a maniac. I refused to answer because I was at the beach and there was no pay phone in sight. When I got home, I saw his shadow and told Myra, he is in here! She asked where, but when I blinked and turned the light on, he was gone. I thought it was my imagination. She walked me in so she could listen to all of the voice messages we knew he left on my answering machine. To our surprise, he had only left one.

I walked her to my door and she was telling me how I need to leave him alone and I agreed. When I locked the door, went upstairs, he come from underneath my bed. I remember him ripping my jacket off, breaking the zipper and telling me he was going to kill me because I ignored him and I did not appreciate him being the only man that would ever love me as fat as I was!

He pretended to have a gun and told me we were going for a ride. My mother had my daughter overnight and I did not want her to come to my home with my daughter only to find me dead, so I went with him. We drove around all night, he cried and begged me to forgive him for paging me all day, he was just scared I was with another man. The whole time he was talking I was praying to get out alive and promising God I would never speak with him again if I just made it home safely.

A normal person would have kept their promise to God, but because I was so overtaken by the FGs, I broke my promise to God. After computer man took me home safely, I lasted about one week before I started answering his calls again. The FGs reminded me to be humble, not to have too much pride and keep ignoring him because after all he was generally a nice guy, plus with him we could eat all we wanted, when we wanted, wherever we wanted. We could eat delicious snacks even when I was not hungry. So I stayed for years, in misery, but the FGs were happy.

Being the middle child, I knew how to adapt. I know how to adjust my mindset to accommodate those around me. I was being guided by the evil FGs and they taught me how to be a fraud to myself. I learned to fake so good, I had myself fooled, then the ultimate happened. The absolute worst experience I had with computer man was when a girlfriend and I wanted to go out but she did not have a babysitter. I asked computer man if he could watch her minor aged daughter since he would be watching his children that night anyway and he agreed. I told my friend and her daughter it was OK. He appeared to be a great father to his children and he interacted very well with my daughter.

When we returned everyone was asleep and the night ended well. So well, that it became a pattern. I was relieved to finally have a friend that computer man would actually suggest I hang out with. If I said my friend did not have money to go out, he would give me enough money for both of us to go and have a good time.

My friend would tell me how lucky I was to have him. The money I earned from working my 9-5, he insisted I only spend on my daughter and my bills.

He always covered my entertainment and personal shopping. After six months of she and I having regular girls nights out at his expense, my friend daughter revealed computer man was molesting her.

My heart stopped, I was sick and never felt so helpless in all of my life. I had no power at all. At first, I was in disbelief because his children never said such a thing, and oh my God, my daughter!! She had never said such a thing. They were never alone, even if my daughter was away with my mother, we only left her daughter when his children were there, so when could this have happened?

After further investigation and hearing the little girl out, I knew without a doubt she was telling the truth. I felt life leave my body. I became numb and cold. My friend wanted to kill him but neither of us wanted to go to prison so we called the police. He was arrested. I forced myself to show up to court for every hearing to be with my friend and her daughter but the pain in her mother's eyes and her eyes took a piece out of me every time I saw them. It was a three-year process and I hated every second but I felt responsible and I had to see justice served.

On one of the last days of me dragging myself to court, I went home only to find all of prized possessions were stolen, except the police would not allow me to report it stolen because the person who stole it had a key to my house. I trusted computer man with keys to my house and he gave the keys to his mother (who admitted to having my stuff). She decided while I was away, to go in and take whatever she wanted including my personal photo albums with all of my daughter's baby photos, my journals, my trophies from when I played softball and basketball, my collectable figurines and more.

I pleaded with her and offered for her to keep the replaceable stuff, just return my photo albums, especially the one with the ultrasound picture of my daughter. She said she would return it if I convinced my friend to drop the charges against her son and I walk away as well. She promised he would not hurt another child. I could not turn my back on justice so I declined her offer. She debated with me, saying I was being dramatic because it was not as if I was physically hurt or my daughter destroyed, she just wanted her son back. I refused and never regained custody of my possessions.

At this time, we were living in a five-bedroom home in Anaheim Hills. I certainly did not need the space but I was sharing responsibilities with someone else, which meant we could afford it so why not? After learning what a creep he was, he went to prison and I let go of the house. Once again, I "gave away" a home and started over. Charity and I moved back in with my parents for a short while, which was a tremendous blessing but also the most humbling experience I have been through.

I went from living on a hill to sharing a twin-size bed with my daughter, sharing a room with my younger sister and my niece. We did not have closet space so I kept our clothes for the week in my car trunk, and all other clothes were stored in my baby niece's closet at my brother and sister-in-love house in Compton. On Sundays, I would have to pray they were available so I could drive to their home and exchange clothes for the following week.

I felt horrible, like a complete failure. When I walked away from the home in Chino, Charity was fairly young, I did not feel like she would notice the difference. Walking away from the house in Anaheim Hills came with her asking why and begging for us to please go back to our house. That experience gave tremendous strength to the FGs. They quietly held on to the power for later use. I continued existing in life, I had to be strong for my daughter, I had to somehow manage to keep up my tough girl image even though I was dying inside.

My family knew about the situation, as did some of my friends, but no one, I believe, understood the pain I was feeling. They only saw my Wonder Woman, superhero shell and ignored me getting bigger and bigger as a sign of a cry for help.
I saw their attitude as if it were saying, "Well, it didn't happen to us so it's all good."

I was breaking inside and no one saw it. When I tried to express my falling apart, all I got was, "You are strong, you will make it through", "Forget about it, move on, this is not your fault", "Well what's your next move", "They didn't steal everything, you still have your clothes". The worst comment of all was, "At least they left your refrigerator".

The photos of my daughter, the trophies I earned were mine, and to me that was everything, but because they left my refrigerator, I was "exaggerating" or being "dramatic" when I said they took everything. I even went to my pastor at church and confided in him, and I will never forget what he said. "Is someone pressing charges against this guy? OK, good. Take care".

I was devastated! I had been a help to so many people and when I felt I was at my wit's end, completely losing it, my only support systems were still counting on me to be the strong one. The only real support I felt I had was my FGs. They never left my side, they even called a few of their friends over to sit with me at night while I cried and ate ice cream.

I put my dating life on hiatus. I gave up. I was surrendering whatever power I thought I had because I wanted to give up, on purpose. I was tired of holding it all together and pretending.

I did not want any power nor to be in control. Being the evil creatures they are, there was no pity, the FGs were still thriving and they were more power hungry than ever. By this time, they had taken control of my mind and they refused to give up power. They displayed their need for power by convincing me to drive to McDonald's and use my power to demand hot and fresh.

I went to Taco Bell and ordered enchiritos, extra sauce, In-N-Out with mustard and grilled onions on my burger. I said it, and they did it. That became a surviving must for the FGs, we were using that power sometimes two or three times a day. It was my only fix so I went with it. I had gone years neglecting myself. My work performance dropped because I was running back and forth to court. When I was not going to court, I was at my desk crying.

I had mastered the art of being selfless, being humble, accepting people from all walks and levels in life into my world. I went out of my way to make sure everyone around me was happy. When I call you a friend, I am that and more, I love hard and I give my all, even if it is hurting me. I never imagined I would ever play a major part in the worst days of a sweet, innocent little girl's life.

Then in 2008, after nine years of working faithfully for Pacificare, where I worked my way up from a helpdesk operator, claims examiner all the way up to being an auditor, I was laid off because they found cheaper labor in Ireland. I was back to being a single mother and I could not be jobless. I was actually happy about being laid off because they were part of my environment that found me running back and forth to court pointlessly.

I was happy to get away from them, but I still stress-ate because they were letting me go. I knew I had to work somewhere. My enemies, the FGs, could not have been happier. They thought this was sending me into a downward spiral. I believe this was when the FGs started to run out of patience. I weighed 132 pounds when I was married at 21, 240 pounds when I delivered my daughter, 145 pounds from age 22 to 30 years old, 185 pounds at 32, 240 at 35 and this was the end point for the FGs.

They no longer wanted to wait for the perfect time. They no longer wanted to slowly creep out. They couldn't take it anymore and were ready to end me. Here I was thinking we had a nice relationship, unknowingly I was welcoming them in my body and allowing them to control me because I accepted them as comforting friends. Before my last day at Pacificare, I received a call from Kaiser Permanente telling me they were hiring and interested in interviewing me. I went in, got the job and was asked to get a physical before I started working.

The physical is when I was faced the truth: My FGs were my enemies. They were evil and they were out to kill me! When I learned they were frauds, I was woke and fully aware of my internal battle, so the real battle began. I knew I had to do something permanent but I did not know how or what. I left the doctor 's office with determination and good thoughts, which was fine by the FGs but they were not giving up on their mission to destroy me.

My first month at Kaiser was spent in Pasadena. I love that city! I could not wait for lunch time to come, not for me to eat but for me to walk down Colorado Boulevard and window shop! I would have a light lunch at the local sushi bar but that was only because the city of Pasadena is also a bit pricey and I did not want to spend $15 a day on lunch.

My walking daily at lunch time was enough to make a difference in my health and enough to alarm the FGs. They were beyond excited when my training was over and I could go to my home office to work daily. My home office included amazing peers. Going to work was like going to hang out with family. I was on a team with seven other people: Jeff, Alex, Salina, Sylvia, Juliana, Christina and Ricardo.

They welcomed me immediately and quickly advised me of our monthly grocery bill of $5 each. Someone would be responsible for collecting the money at the beginning of each month and going to Costco for "office food", which mainly consisted of Cup O Noodles, chips, cookies, and sweetened Kool-Aid powder. They were veterans on the job so they often left and went out to the field. I, on the other hand, sat in the office self-learning our product and having access to snacks all day!

My favorite snack was to fill my cup with crushed ice from the hospital cafeteria and sprinkle sweetened Kool- Aid powder over the ice. After a minute or so, it transformed into the most delicious slushy in the world. I was not attentive to all of the sugar I was consuming all day long!

Even after snacking all morning, when my fifth hour of work came around, the FGs would trigger my brain and convince me it was eating time. I would get in my car and drive to a fast food place to eat. My office was in a prime location because just about whatever you desired to eat was less than five minutes away.

Unlike Pasadena, food was affordable and most places gave a hospital discount, to make the gluttony more tempting. After the second year of working with morning donuts, snacking, office pizza parties, potlucks, I was up to 250 pounds. Ironically, it seems as if I was the only one who gained weight, my peers remained the same size, if not smaller. I recognized that I was the only one under attack and even questioned myself about my decisions, yet I allowed the FGs to still deceive me. This is how I know the FGs are out to get me. I am their special mission!

TT*:* I wonder if I was not forced to eat everything on my plate as a child if I would be in this struggle today. Growing up I did not have the option to say I am not hungry now, or that is too much food on my plate. Rather, I was told when eating time was, regardless if I was hungry or not. I was commanded to eat everything on my plate at every meal. That is the reason I am the way I am. I know I am not hungry but because California law says I have to take a lunch break no later than 12 p.m. I seem to always eat at 12 p.m. So what if I just had a hearty breakfast at 9 a.m. I abide by the rules because I was raised to abide by the rules. If my parent or guardian deemed it to be eating time, then it was eating time. It has become an awful habit.

FGs: "Good work, let's keep her in that frame of mind. It is her disciplined upbringing that is causing her to eat unnecessarily. We know that is not the case, just because the clock says it is "lunch time" does not mean it is 'eating time'. She is an adult now and can read a book on her determined lunch time and eat a salad or a sandwich when she is really hungry. She does not work in a controlled environment that dictates where and what she eats, but as long as she thinks she is 'obeying' the rules, we have her in the palms of our hands."

We were an awesome team but just like everything else in life, things must change. Jeff, Salina, Alex and Sylvia took on positions in different departments, Juliana and Christina moved out of state, and unfortunately Ricardo passed away. I received a new team of people and although great, none could ever replace my home team. The new crew was just as friendly but came in with their own mind-sets.

We worked as a team but not a unit. The Costco runs ended because things became too difficult, some people had to be gluten free, others no peanuts. One girl would literally carry one red apple around with her all day in case she got hungry because that was the only thing she would allow herself to eat all day. She said when we are working we should only focus on work, not food and breaks. She only had the apple to prevent her from fainting from hunger. She could carry that apple for days without taking a bite.

Other people obsessed over whether they looked fat or not because the scale read 108 pounds that morning when they promised themselves never to go over 105 pounds. Some would come to work after going to the gym and skipping a shower. They would rather smell like dog sweat at work then risk losing an ounce of muscle mass. Even the men were difficult. They would debate whether they should grow a beard or not because the extra hair on their face might make them look fat. They would discuss how they hadn't eaten bread in months or eaten from a fast food place in years.

I would listen to the conversations and literally want to throw everyone out the window. Their care for health was a bit too extreme for me. The FGs couldn't wait for me to get away from them so I could be alone with junk food. Cheetos, Toblerone candy and Cactus Coolers were great stress relievers and made the FGs extremely happy but never satisfied! Looking back, I feel like all of their food and weight phobias were because of my size. No one ever said anything flat out to my face, but if you pay attention, people 's actions will speak a thousand words.

Maybe if I had taken heed of some of their words, I would have changed my mindset about some of my food choices. The FGs had convinced me that they were annoying and pathetic. There were so many more problems in life to deal with and they chose to stress over grams of sugar in a can of Coke.

I would leave work mentally drained. Being the veteran on the team, I was looked at by management to be a leader when it came to work. After listening to the "Oh my God do I look fat, I should not have eaten three Tic Tacs" conversations, I had to force myself to respond kindly and without disgust when I heard the same voices asking me work-related questions.

I take great pride in my work so I always gave them my best but that was draining and I needed an outlet! The FGs stay on alert and being that they are the author of confusion and deception, and if we are not very careful and aware, they will take something good and trick us into allowing it to become something bad. I was seeking a "healthy" outlet when the next opportunity appeared in my life, which was perfect timing for the FGs to utilize their cleverness and use my ignorance to their advantage.

Fate reacquainted me with Juaquin Hawkins, an old high school peer who would introduce me to the next chapter of my life that utilized my God-given talents. Trained to not want the spotlight, always wanting the best for others, it was a no brainer when I was asked to represent Juaquin, aka "Hawk". He is a friend and I could help tell his story. It was my pleasure and it worked for both of us because he gained a loyal, trustworthy advocate and I gained a constructive way to occupy my time outside of work in corporate America. The FGs used this as a weapon, because they figured they would distract me from killing them because my mind would be occupied with learning a new role outside of healthcare and starting a new business venture. I would never have time or energy for a gym or to even eat home cooked meals regularly. In 2010, I founded T.C.P.R. (Tonya Carmouche Public Relations), a small public relations boutique.

Chapter Five

The ~~Steaks~~ Stakes Are Higher

Starting Tonya Carmouche Public Relations (TCPR) was perfect for me. I embarked upon a role that would allow me to help others achieve their dreams, build success and make money. I quickly became one of the best because I did not want the shine, I made sure clients always came first. The FGs had me believing I was doing a great service by helping everyone else with their vision but not having a real vision of my own, I wanted the best for everyone and did not think of me.

My first clients included a multi-cultural girls singing group, a child rapper from Compton, a former producer from Death Row records, and of course my former NBA player, Hawk. I was so focused on getting my boutique off the ground, I would spend my lunch breaks making phone calls and following up on emails. I would often walk on my lunch break to clear my mind of medical stuff and allow PR thoughts and ideas to come in.

This became a conflict of interest for the FGs because my new distraction was causing me to neglect them. Focused on starting my own business, I was unintentionally losing weight. Randomly and out of the blue, one day I was invited to be in a Kaiser ad! After the ad came out, the FGs were talking:

FGs: "Guys, have you seen the Kaiser ad that has Tonya photos displaying 'healthy' living? She even became an ambassador for their wellness program. All because she lost 60 of us! We should be concerned guys, this could be the very thing that keeps her on track this time! We know image is everything to her these days. If all eyes are on her, she may stay focused. We have to do something!"

TT: Now that I am an ambassador, I have to keep my determination going. My new look will also help me in my PR world.

FGs: "Let's convince Kaiser to not use her photos after all, or if they do use them put them in Colorado or anywhere she will hopefully never see. This way she won't be reminded constantly that she almost conquered us. If she sees herself successful on a regular basis, she will stay pumped. We have to get in her head and make her think her victory was for naught, it was a temporary win and not worth the work." This was a short-lived lifestyle. The more my PR clientele picked up, the more time I had to spend working on my lunch break. I had to schedule calls before work or during my break/lunch time so I could go to my car for a quiet environment. Before long the FGs had gotten to me again. After lunch, I would feel like I was starving, literally like I would faint if I did not eat something immediately.

TT: I will have to cut my calls a tad bit shorter so I can go for fast food from one of the many locations surrounding my office. Besides, the only people around me that saw my Kaiser ad were those I showed the photo proofs that were sent to me. It was not like I was up on a billboard around the facility I worked at, so no one would recognize me for being the Health Ambassador anyway. I was back to snacking at my desk and developed worse habits than before. I knew weight was a problem for me but was not noticing the FGs slowly creeping back up on me. I was still working corporate successfully and developing a booming company. I felt just fine.

FGs: "We got her in a good spot guys. She has the mindset that she is just fine, she is not as bad off as other people. We know she is well on the road to arriving to where we want her to be, if we just keep her unaware, we will succeed."

My PR boutique continued to grow and I continued accepting clients who had little or no name recognition, nor did they have money to pay me. I let the fact that I didn't go to school for PR put little value on myself, despite me having three degrees in other subjects, including a Master's degree.

I had very low esteem when it came to PR, so I often worked with no pay and was OK with it because

I felt I was learning. I accepted random stipends and did not complain because I figured I was new to the game and didn't have much experience. I worked a full-time job and I could only dedicate my break time and after hours to clients. I did not realize I was not valuing my worth, but the FGs did and they took advantage of every chance they had.

I wanted all of my clients to succeed so I ran to every event, stood on every red carpet, wrote every press release. My path was tough because I had to become super creative to get media, event planners and other PR peers to accept my clients.

I sacrificed and did not mind it at all. I went to events when I wanted to work out. I deprived myself of sleep because I was always up early calling people on the East Coast at their 8 a.m. hour (5 a.m. for me), and I was up late at night either writing or attending an event. I was stopping by fast food places late at night because I no longer had time to cook homemade meals. That meant I was eating fast food for lunch and dinner. The FGs loved it.

After a year of grinding and gaining, I attracted a few name clients. They would comment on how impressive my hustle was and they wanted to come aboard. Still being focused on wanting the best for others, accommodating others at all times, I gave my best. Everyone was amazed at how far I had come.

I was booking clients on syndicated radio shows that ranked number one on major stations, I was booking clients appearances on televised award shows, had clients featured in award-winning published magazines found in Barnes & Noble, Target, Wal-Mart and other shopping outlets, clients sung national anthems in historic arenas, I fought for opportunities to get my clients in front of hundreds of thousands of people solely based on their work from the past.

I taught myself how to make yesterday's news appealing in the present day. I booked so many interviews, I lost count. I was introducing clients to potential investors for their projects, and I was working for little or no pay.

Imagine the slap in the face I felt when people started thanking me and telling me I had outworked their previous well-known publicist and many other publicists they know who were paid $800-$2,000 a month! I have the propensity to win or at least appear as a winner. I was so busy making sure I was a success I neglected me, again. Being in the PR business gave me great joy, I truly loved doing it and enjoyed the opportunities that I had to create for others, I appreciated the power I felt when things went well.

When things did not go so well, it became a different story. I had to work even more to try to keep my clients relevant. There were so many days where I was overwhelmed with frustration because of all of the "No, we are not interested" answers I would receive over and over again. The "nos" opened the door for the FGs to reign over my weight-loss accomplishments. When the FGs noticed the toll the "nos" were taking on me, I found myself being placed in a position of receiving more no's than ever.

I started falling out of love with PR. I was feeling beat up, used and abused. I was unhappy. The more unhappy I was, the more I ate, and the more I ate the more unhappy I became. It was a vicious cycle that the FGs had a ball with. I was doing everything, a one woman show, and little or no appreciation was shown. When I would book an appearance or interview, it felt like I had to beg them to show up and participate. It was as if they expected me to deliver more than I was. I never told them about all I was doing for their career, they certainly did not know about all of the "no's". That may have crushed them. Instead, I carried the burden alone.

I caught myself and thought, "This has to stop. I am not getting anywhere and I am feeling like I am believing in other people's dreams more than they do themselves." I had to do a roster sweep and let go of the clients that were completely draining me or I felt I could no longer be of service to without causing myself harm. Some clients chose to leave and take on "Beverly Hills" publicists. That baffled me because if they could not afford to pay me even gas money, how could they afford Beverly Hills?

I later saw them without representation and realized they had gotten caught up in fantasy land thinking others would work for free as I had. They were put to the curb immediately. I was not into PR for the money. I was always honest and sincerely wanted the best for everyone. I served my clients from a place of passion, belief and love.

That is what made me unique. Hollywood is funny, but that is another story. The clients I have now know the work I put in for them and they appreciate what I do. They stuck by my side and taught me that not everyone is a puppet for the FGs. These people are genuine, I love them and respect their craft. Even after my roster sweep and only keeping a handful of clients who have become my extended family, the FGs still managed to allow to use any excuse not to focus on me. I would say I did not have time, I was traveling, I stayed on the grind so eating junk fueled me. I solved problems all day, I should not have to think about what to eat that is healthy. The FGs would tell me to treat myself to Starbucks since I could not afford Gucci.

The FGs took seven consecutive years to shine and do tons of damage. After juggling and rearranging my PR boutique, all original 60 managed to return with even more friends. I felt like I went from small to Biggie Smalls overnight (minus the checks). Then I had another wakeup call. One day when I was feeling really great I was speaking with my friend Laura who happens to be a RN when randomly we decided to take my blood pressure. The look on her face was scary! She sent me right away to see a doctor.

TT: The doctor was right all along, you guys are trying to kill me. I had my blood pressure checked today and it was 168/98. I was being asked questions such as, "Are you dizzy, do you feel faint, do you have headaches"? I was scared! Thanks to you FGs I have to take medications now without skipping a day. I can't do this back and forth relationship anymore. God help me! I can do all things through Christ that strengthens me. My body is the dwelling temple of the living God. Greater is He that is in me than he that is in the world. No temptation has overtaken me except what is common to mankind. God is faithful. He will not let me be tempted beyond what I can bear, but when I am tempted He will also provide a way out so I can endure it!

FGs: "Now she is quoting scriptures and pulling on her real inner strength. Looks like our jig is up. Let's make a deal with her. Hey, TT, how about we allow 50 or 60 of us to leave your body and let you live 10 more years than we initially were? In return, you continue to feed us junk, not exercise and we both continue to feel loved and happy. One thing. If we spare your life, we at least have to cause you knee and back pain for the rest of your life, after all, we have hung in here for years and worked hard to destroy you, you can let us have a little success, right? At least you won't have to make big changes."

Chapter 6

The 6-foot Candy Bar

Home stretch

The day I went to visit my doctor for a normal checkup and physical, I was warned by the physician that Fat Genes are known to be sheep in wolves' clothing. They pretend to be the ultimate comforter when all along they are plotting and planning to perform a homicide on their naive mate. I was in disbelief! After a failed marriage, building friendships over the years that ended abruptly, deaths in the family, being laid off from work, the Fat Genes seemed to be the only constant in my life.

Never once did they complain about their dwelling place, never once did they leave me feeling unloved and alone, that was not an event that was experienced once. "They want to kill me? No, surely this person in a white coat must be a hater. How dare he suggest we break up!"

I had already tried telling myself that the FGs had to go based on my personal frustrations and vanity alone, but now that I had a medical doctor telling me they were planning to kill me, I was beyond angry. I was pissed off and embarrassed. I have to now take medication because I allowed myself to be manipulated by FGs for years. These sneaky FGs literally drove me to eat my way into high blood pressure! Holding true to character, the FGs quickly invaded my thoughts and convinced me that the doctor was overreacting! It is his job to scare patients and push prescription drugs, this is how he gets paid the big bucks.

I immediately called my mother and shared this awful advice I received and mother agreed with the doctor. I thought: "No, no, no, this can't be, who will love me"? I could tell I had gained weight but I was still cute, at least I felt. In addition, I felt fine. I was still running around with my daughter, I was still hanging out with friends, men were still hitting on me, heck, I even had a woman hit on me, I was not this obese creature the doctor was making me out to be.

That night I went to visit my best friend, Myra, and again I shared the information. Myra suggested changing my eating habits a little bit and maybe the Fat Genes would go back in hiding for another 30 years.
I finally agreed, and this is where my relationship with the FGs turned into a personal WWIII. My sincerity with myself kicked the FGs into street dirty fighting mode.

The FGs were not giving up that quickly, they convinced me to go home, eat a great meal, because after all, I would be eating less and more healthy starting tomorrow so I had to get it all in that night. In the morning, I stood naked, looking in the mirror, pulling the excess fat all over my body and visualizing the alien FGs. I started a conversation with them:

TT: Good morning, FGs. Today is the beginning of a new us. I will not feed you a muffin and Frappuccino from Starbucks for breakfast today, we will not have Cheetos for a mid-morning snack, we will not have McDonald's for lunch, and certainly we will not have chili-cheese fries from Louis Burgers for dinner. I will still feed you. So please do not feel I am neglecting you. Instead, we will have oatmeal for breakfast, apple for snack, El Pollo for lunch, almonds for late day snack, and baked chicken for dinner. Sounds good right? RIGHT?

FGs: "Is she serious? She is going to listen to those haters!! Those lonely, pathetic creatures, she is going to play us for them? She loves us, she will be back to treating us right, let's just hold our ground."

TT: It's been a month, so far the change is OK, I am being healthier, and FGs are still here with me. I've noticed some have started being timid, hiding in their secret spot they lived in for years.

FGs: "It's been a month and she is still trippin'! We have to stand strong, we have to remain a unit. The 10 of you that have become these timid infants, shrinking and hiding, MAN UP, get back out here. We have to be strong, she loves us so much she is not going to believe the truths the doctor told her. Sure, we are planning to kill her, but not for another 10 years at least. She was supposed to never question our motive. She was supposed to keep being ignorant to the importance of health. LOOK, LOOK, she is in See's Candies!! Please let there be a sale, please let the sales lady give her a sample that will snap her back to the oblivious state she was content with."

TT: Speaking to the See's sales clerk, "Um, no thank you, I will pass on the sample. I need to just pick up a gift for a friend. Oh, really, it's the new flavor, only for a season? Oh, in that case, yes, I will try it." Thinking to myself, FGs, hope you like this treat because after the season I can't feed you this kind again. After the sales clerk handed me the sample, I said, "Thank you" and thought, oh my goodness it seem like forever since I felt this way. I turned to the sales clerk and said "OK, OK, I will buy a pound, but only because this kind will soon be going away soon."

FGs: "HA HA HA, told yall!! This feels good, we are getting our energy back, so what if it is draining all of her energy. We are up and running, come on troops let's race to her brain and make her think she is still hungry. On the mark, set, go!! LOOK, LOOK, LOOK, this is amazing, we are at the Taco Bell drive-through. Hello little Taco Bell dog, we missed seeing your picture weekly."

Three months later

TT: Forget the dumb advice of depriving myself to be healthy, going to bed with hunger pangs, feeling empty. That's the pits. I will finish out this year, and then torture myself in January! Here ya go, FGs, have some Cold Stones, you like that huh? I can tell, you are making me feel tingly inside, I'm smiling again. I see you all have returned. Some of you are even bolder. You really want to be seen this time, huh? Guess I will go buy bigger clothes so everyone can be comfortable.

Six months later

As I sat at my desk feeling numb on the right side, I was thinking to myself, this does not feel right. I better go see the doctor. My right arm and fingers are numb, what's up?

TT: Oh man, here we go again! He just said it was your fault FGs, he is sending me down for MRIs but he is certain it is all your fault. My God, could the doctor have been telling the truth? FGs are you trying to kill me??? Wow, I am offended, really you guys!

Running around so much you've caused my blood pressure to be high. You've even attacked my cholesterol level? I thought you loved me. You are breaking my heart, LITERALLY, you heard the doctor, he said you were very close to giving me a heart attack... (crying) How could you? That's it, guys. It's over. I will never feed you how you like again, from now on it is all on my terms. I chose to make my terms equivalent to the physician's.

TT: "Aw, man, see I told you just do it at once, BAM!! She would not know what hit her. Y'all wanted to do it slow, well did we forget she works in a hospital now and would run to one of her doctor friends at the first sign of something going wrong? Now we have made her mad. She is going to make us eat that boring food again. Good news is, it won't last long. OK, here is the plan, she is going to eat healthier for a few months, 30 of us will shrink back, and give her the illusion she is all right. We will be back at Fat Burger in no time."

A year later:

FGs: "See, told you we should have took her out early, she is still eating blasted garlic baked chicken. What happened to the month? Heck, we were still strong at six months, but a year? REALLY. Hey, hey, where are you guys going? My front line 60 get back here, NOW!! Of course she is not serious, this is just a longer phase. We have to stay strong. Come on guys... guys, guys, why are you leaving? Why do you have a U-Haul? You moving out forever? Wait, wait, wait, we cannot break up this unit. We back to being 100 strong, we must remain 100.

Come back, come back. WELL BYE THEN. I am glad you're leaving forever!! Ok, 40, it is just us now, hold on, she will give in soon. we have to remain, we have been here for so long, we are comfortable, we have raised our children, seen them off to college, we have built pools that are flowing with Wesson oil, we will have grandchildren living in other bodies, we have retired, and now all we have to do is plainly live off the fat of our land, the little that is left. We have been here so long, we are only familiar with her. She will be back, watch and see."

TT: I am getting on this treadmill today, I don't care how tired I am!

FGs: "Make her favorite Carmouche cousin, Darrin, call her. She will stop this treadmill crap and speak with him."

TT: Dang it D, why are you calling now? I have to get this workout in, I will call you later.

FGs: "Oh, what? She ignored Darrin? She never ignores him! Guys, this is really bad!! We have to do something to make her regret not putting off her silly treadmill run!"

TT: How could this be? Why was Darrin calling me? I cannot believe he flipped his truck over on the 110 freeway and left this life. Oh my God, if I could only go back to that day, I would have taken his phone call. I will never forgive myself. I love him...

FGs: "Got her..."

TT: Darrin always encouraged me to go to Planet Fitness with him, only we would end up getting a hydro massage, leaving and going to Chipotle. We never worked out. I will honor him and do what we should have been doing all along, continue to go to the gym but I will actually workout. I will continue my healthy mission. I will remember the many, many great times and laughs we shared. I will forever hold his secrets. I will cherish him and continue striving for greatness, I know he would have been proud.

FGs: "Wait, what?"

In a year, I had managed to lose 60 pounds. I cut out mostly all junk food, I walked 4 miles a day twice a week and rode my bike 5 miles three times a week. I dropped all energy drinks, I stopped entertaining dating because it seemed as if I was only attracting losers. I had complete focus.

TT: Come on FGs, all of you have to leave. I don't love you anymore, and I have found comfort in other things. Exercise, movies, concerts, reading, and networking have all embraced me. I am happy with just me, I don't need you. JUST GO already. I have tried running you out, walking you out, biking you out, dancing you out, and Zumba. Why won't you leave? I don't want you. I know you hate me, I know you want to kill me, so go. There is nothing you can do to make me give in to you. You guys were trying to leave my daughter motherless, that is the ultimate. I will never comfort you again. I see you for the wolves you are.

FGs: "Troops, she is serious this time. We put a humongous guilt trip on her after the death of her cousin, and she shook it off. We have been to parties, through holidays, several stressful situations and she has not budged. Sure, she samples here and there but that is it a sample. We need more and she is not giving in. Oh man, we are doomed.

All the water she has been drinking has ruined our pools, and what is with her taking all of our energy? She already walked 3 miles today, why is she getting on a bike? This heifer has lost her mind. We are getting weak guys, we have to hold on. Stop crying, where are you going? Why are you standing at the door with a suitcase? Come on, come on. Has anyone heard from the 60? Really, they found a new home and they are at Rocky Mountain Chocolate Factory right now? We love that place, but this new Donna Richardson wannabe won't take us. How dare she eat a measly tootsie roll and say this is enough. She has really lost her rabbit mind, a tootsie roll. She can play dirty if she wants, we are staying. Let the weak say we strong, let me hear it? Hello? Guys, come on, we have to stay!!"

TT: OK, you last 40, I have a surprise for you this month. Jump rope. I will shake rattle and roll you off. Surely, you will be gone by the beginning of the year. And, oh yes, since you want to be so stubborn, there will be no more tootsie rolls for the month of October. I told you once I saw your true colors and it was a done deal. You are not welcomed anymore. And, yes, that is an exercise ball I just purchased. Then he came...Another friend from high school. I call him Major. He was a real-life man-child who dragged me right back to the gutter of obesity and gave the FGs the upper hand.

At first, it was great. It all started with complete innocence, I was honestly only helping him, a friend.

He was going through a really rough time in his life and I offered my assistance. I treated him how I imagined I would have liked to be treated if I was in the same situation. Unfortunately, he did not treat me in return in a way I would have treated someone being a friend to me and that triggered me to letting my guard down and the FGs to rule my life once again.

It started with sitting with him at the hospital with one of his parents. I would drive 45 minutes in traffic, sometimes more, almost daily to just sit with him and let him know he was not alone. I would go after work and arrive close to 7 p.m. After sitting and talking for awhile, we would go grab food, come back, sit and talk some more. I would get home around 11 p.m., wide awake because of my adrenaline being high out of concern for his family.

When I did finally fall asleep, it always felt like moments before the alarm went off for me to go to the office again for work. After the need for us to hang out at the hospital was over, he started coming by my place. I would cook most nights and we would eat and watch movies. I was president of a non-profit at the time so we would also brainstorm on ways to help the organization. He did not have a car so I would have to drive him home every night, causing me to miss out on much-needed sleep, but I did not complain and the FGs loved every moment because they knew after I took him home, I would come back to clean the kitchen and most times eat again, and it was too late to be even tasting food.

After several months, I was burnt out on the driving back and forth, so I welcomed the nights where he would fall asleep on the downstairs sofa and I could get a few hours of rest before I started work again. By the end of the year, Major had managed to become a full-time house guest. We never had a discussion or an agreement, the sofa just became his permanent sleeping spot. I wanted him to leave but he was a friend and I did not know how to say it, especially after hearing him constantly say he had nowhere else to go. Having Major living with me appeared as if I had a live-in lover who was helping me with my bills and causing my life to become better. That was not the case at all, in fact, having him living with me introduced me to a level of stress I will never live through again. We never kissed, hugged or even held hands. He never spoke of any responsibilities or had conversations of substance. Instead, he was just there, my instant problem child.

He refused to work, never had any money, ate more than me, always needed a ride somewhere, was messy, did not do chores, could not help with the yard because of asthma, had the communication skills of a cotton ball, no drive, no joy, just nothing, but I called him friend and I endured. The FGs were fully awakened and came back with a vengeance. They convinced me to drink energy drinks, chips, candy all day everyday so I could have energy to cook, clean, work a second job, and maintain a household that now included a daughter and an adult "son".

The years went by extremely fast. Before I knew it, three years had passed. I didn't notice the FGs taking over because several times a week, he would borrow my vehicle and "forget" I got off work at 5 p.m., causing me to walk home. I could have taken an Uber or Lyft but I lived less than two miles from my office so I walked and the FGs made me think that this would balance out the chili cheese fries, fried chicken, candy, pie, chips and soda I had consumed while at work.

During the third year, I was sued by a credit company and lost. The ruling was to take $1,000 out of my paycheck each month until my debt was paid in full. I told Major and being the man-child he is, his reply was, "That's illegal, no one can do that!" When I opened my check that month, sure enough it was negative $1,000. I told Major, "I don't have money for gas, food, I barely have enough to keep a roof over our head." Just like with my ex-husband and almost everyone else in my life, his final reply was, "Well what will you do?".

He never said don't worry, you carried me for years, I will make sure we have lights, gas, and food. Instead, he said, "Well, we don't need to eat. We can both lose some weight." That statement caused the FGs to turn on him and slap some sense into my brain.

FGs: "Wait a minute, we encouraged TT to provide shelter, transportation, food, toiletries, clothes, Internet, cable, cell phone, entertainment, and a bucket list of other stuff for this bum all in the name of friendship and he is refusing to inconvenience himself to go earn enough money to feed us a measly peanut butter and jelly sandwich? He must go!" I woke up one day with the determination he had to leave. I gave him a two-week notice to get out. On days he would try to be considerate by cooking something I managed to purchase with my money, I would think, "Well, maybe he is trying."

The FGs would instantly kick in and remind me, I went to work and earned the money for this food, I went to work and earned the money to keep the electricity on, I picked up second jobs to earn money to purchase more than Top Ramen, and after he cooks, he will NOT clean so that I don't have to do chores late at night. All this after I have worked all day in the office and after hours at my second job.

When I would look at him and think, "He looks so pathetic, I have to help him", the FGs would kick in and point out, "He's not that cute, he certainly is not your man, he does not care for you or about you. Plus, he refuses to even think of a way to feed us. He must go!"

The FGs were upset because he was dipping into their fast food and Starbucks money. I had enough and finally threatened him to leave. I had written an eviction letter (although he never paid a dime on any bill), waited a month and informed him I would be dropping all of his belongings off in front of his parents' old house (the last known address I knew for him). I didn't care who lived there, they were walking up to a trash bag of his belongings. He threw his stuff in a yard-size trash bag and left. I had my play brother Van come immediately over and change my locks.

Major was a drastic pitfall but the FGs were at their wits' end with me losing them, so they pulled out all stops with him. The FGs played on my emotions and even on my "Christianity" by making me believe I was being Christ-like and helping my fellow man in need. Then the FGs kept me blinded when I took my Christ-like behavior and turned myself into Major's personal Christ, forsaking myself and providing for his needs. Never again. After walking away from him, I thought back on how many other times I had changed my plans to accommodate others at the expense of my life. I am dependable and that attracts people to me. I was not a "yes" person because if I could absolutely not do something I would say "no" and have no regrets. I just didn't like letting people down, so nine times out of 10 I found a way to say yes.

If I had plans to work out after work but someone needed to vent after work over drinks, I changed MY plans. If I had plans to work out before work but someone wanted to text early morning about their boyfriend problems, I changed MY plans and stayed in bed texting them back. If I planned on cooking at home but someone wanted to go to happy hour for wings because they did not feel like cooking, I changed MY plans and met up with them. I did whatever I could to make everyone happy except myself.

That is why today I am so very careful about who I allow in my circle. I no longer call everyone a "friend" because I know the personal convictions I have to my friends and the depth I will go to ensure their happiness. I now call people "acquaintances", "clients", "peers", "that guy", "her", anything to keep my mindset within boundaries. Some people may be offended and I am OK with that. The FGs tried to remind me of my "Imitation of Life" perception fear and I had to shake that thought off. Think of me as you may, I have to live for me.

I've learned from that experience that I have to be extremely careful about who I allow to become too close to me. If I see a pattern of drama, a series of bad luck, negative words in every conversation, them entertaining others with no ambition in their life, or they are constantly looking for something to stress over or cry about, I have to keep a distance from them. Otherwise my DNA makeup will cause me to want to "save" them and I will end up giving power to the FGs and killing myself. This was the last inning for the FGs. Just like they had had enough, I had had enough. I am always on alert now watching for their little sneaky ways to trap me again so they can live.

When I got rid of Major I was back to 250 pounds.

Chapter Seven

Flashbacks of the Sabotage

The Real Aha Moment

One day while meditating, I begin to replay in my mind all of the times I spoke of health or leaned towards being healthy and each time I recalled, I envisioned the FGs discussing a way to sabotage my plans. It was surreal to me because I clearly remembered each moment and it felt as if I could actually playback and hear my attempted thoughts and also the sabotaging, influential words of the FGs:

TT: I will shop for healthier food choices and order off the light menu when I go out to eat, that will help me.

FGs: "We know she is a frugal shopper so let's help her do "our" math. Convince her that the cost preparing healthy meals at home can be expensive, then put in her mind that she hates leftovers and after eating the same thing for dinner one night and lunch the next day, she will trash the remaining, thus making her feel bad for wasting money. Now, bombard her mind with commercials and billboards showing her she can get a hamburger, chicken sandwich, fries, cookie and a coke for only $5. Or she can get a chicken breast, potato wedges, biscuit, coleslaw and coke for $5. Better yet, because we know she loves Mexican food, she can get a burrito, a gorgita, nachos, a taco and a Pepsi for $5. For kicks, lets show her she can choose four items from a variety of garbage for $4. She will allow for her brain to wrap around spending $4 or $5 on unhealthy options easier than accepting to pay $30 on the same ol' same. "Our" math makes sense, but if she ever sat down and did the real math, she would ignore our cravings. The real math is sure she is saving $20 today but when we give her the heart attack and the medical bills are thousands of dollars, she will spend far more than the cost of a salad today. It would behoove her to invest in her health voluntarily rather than forcefully to save her life."

TT: If I snack during the day and just eat a fast food value meal at night, I will be able to maintain my weight and not allow any more fat genes into my body. That should be OK.

FGs: "That is OK according to "our" math. What she is failing to realize is even if she eats only 400 extra calories a day, she will gain 2-3 pounds every two weeks. We waited almost 40 years to come out full force, we can be patient and bring our guys back two at a time."

TT: There was a lady on the television saying people stared at her like she was a circus clown. I heard a man say children would point and laugh at him. I read of a lawsuit where a woman was suing because she got fired from her job because of her weight. I see

overweight people sitting alone because they say others are disgusted to sit with them. I never experienced that!
Certainly, I must be fine. I won't go organic and healthy just yet, I'll eat the $5 meals and use my money to pay off bills or something.

FGs: "Well guys, just as planned, we all are back where we belong and we have expanded, let us all welcome the 10 new FGs that have joined us."
TT: I cannot believe myself. Why did I let this happen again? Sure, I can blame work, being a single parent, stress of bills, death in the family, I could say a bunch of stuff but in reality, those excuses are just stuff and lame excuses. I have to take care of me first and stop this from happening. I have the power to do so! I will get back in the gym today!
FGs: "We just overheard her on the phone saying she is going to the gym. Here we go again! Let's get her friend to call her and distract her."
TT: (answering the phone) No, I cannot go to happy hour with you today, so what if it is Taco Tuesday, I am going to the gym. Oh, you want to come to the gym with me? Sure.
FGs: "We chose the wrong friend to have call! Did you hear how easy it was for her to change her mind from going to happy hour to going to the gym with TT? We have to do something before this becomes a daily habit, friends do not hang out at the gym! We know her friend does not want to work out, let's go with that angle."

TT: (greeting her friend), Hey, so glad you could make it. I am on a healthy journey, you are welcome to join me anytime. I am getting on the treadmill now.
FGs: "Look at her walking, make her friend have a cramp! It worked, TT saw her friend in pain and suggested they stop walking. Now they are sitting idle on the stationary bikes discussing reality TV, perfect! That was easy guys. Fifteen more minutes of this and you know TT will be bored and want to leave… and there she goes, walking out of the gym and did not break a sweat! Perfect."
TT: FGs, I know you sent her my way. OK, you got me. I will not invite my friends to work out with me anymore, I will go solo so I can focus. In fact, I will change gym membership and go to the one closer that is on my way home from the office. That way I can start then. That will be perfect because they are always empty around 6 p.m.
FGs: "Guess that was too obvious, maybe we should have invited another friend. She said she will change gyms now, ha, ha, that's an easy fix. Let's make sure everyone in the neighborhood around the gym gets a flyer promoting open enrollment for new members and they can join for free and pay only ten dollars a month for membership!"
TT: What in the world? Why is there suddenly no parking at this gym? For the last year, every time I drove past this gym there were at least 20 empty parking spaces. I am not about to drive around a

parking lot for 30 minutes looking for a parking space, especially after a long day in the office!
FGs: "Where is she going now? The track, oh no guys, it is baseball season, she will get to the track and walk the duration of baseball practice at the college. We have to do something fast, we learned in the past that her walking just for 30 minutes a day will run some of us away."
TT: This is a beautiful day to be walking, I should have been doing this. Fresh air, the sound of bats cracking the ball, this is awesome, except for that man across the street on his lawnmower. That thing is loud and distracting. I have walked the track twice and he is still mowing, will he finish already? Oh great, he just stopped, but why do I still hear the motor buzzing?
FGs: "Who put that Japanese beetle on her shoulder? Hilariously brilliant! That will scare her and she will not come back to the track for months. She sees it, she is running like a mad woman, flying her arms all over the place. Look, she just ran through the baseball field during practice, lol, it worked!! She is getting in her car and leaving, mission accomplished."
TT: This is ridiculous! Two months have passed since I last worked out. I don't want to go to the track anymore because its infested with beetles and flying creatures, I stopped going to the gym because now it seems as if it takes me more time to find a parking space then I am actually in the gym. I need to just get a jump rope and go outside in my own yard. So what if

neighbors are watching! After that, I will go for a walk around my neighborhood.

FGs: "Did everyone hear what she is thinking about doing? She wants to utilize her surroundings, silly woman, we will not let her get rid of us, why does she keep trying! She is saying she wants to do all of this stuff to get rid of us, but look deep into her thoughts, she does not really want to let us go! She is comfortable with us so we just have to keep putting hurdles in her way until she accepts that she is comfortable with us. Look, she is jump-roping now, who does she think she is, a welterweight champion boxer training for the next big fight? Let's get a cat to come stare at her, we know she is afraid of cats. Then when she goes for a walk around the neighborhood, let's use our energy to attract stray dogs to walk with her, that will freak her out for sure! Whoever convinced the bee to follow her while she was walking down the street was brilliant! She was flailing her arms like a wild woman at the bee but people driving by could not see the bee so it just appeared as if she was a crazy person on the loose, that was classic. TT needs to learn we are not going anywhere. Keep the shenanigans coming guys."

TT: I'll buy a treadmill and put it smack in the middle of my living room and I will get up at 6 a.m. to work out or after work for sure

FGs: "Let's make sheets extra soft and warm every morning. She will not get out of bed. After work, lets distract her with work, TV, phone calls, invites, work activities. That treadmill will just be a piece of furniture in no time."

TT: OK, it has been a month since I worked out, I cannot let the FGs keep defeating me. Why do I keep allowing myself to be sidetracked, time is passing by and I am still in the same position I have been in, for years. I know what the issue is so I need to focus. When I am out watering my grass there isn't a cat in sight, the moment I go to exercise, cats want to come and watch me. I know it is the FGs sending them because the cats have a devilish smirk as they intently watch me. Oh, and so much for my walking around the neighborhood! There seems to be a loose dog on every corner, not little dogs, big scary dogs, yet when I am driving through the neighborhood there is never a dog in sight unless it is on a leash with its owner walking it. I have to do something. In the meantime, I will just go back to changing my eating habits.

FGs: "Seems like she is getting "serious" again, we need to do something. Look at her walking to Subway so she can "eat fresh". Let's trip her!"

TT: What in the world? How did I trip over thin air? Unbelievable, I literally tripped over nothing. I bust my lip, hurt my wrist, hurt my leg, have blood hematomas and now I am being told to take it easy from exercising. How could this have happened?

FGs: "Great job, fellas! Some of us actually felt bad for a moment when we saw how hard she hit the ground. We thought for sure she would have knocked a tooth out, but then that would have stopped her from eating and feeding us so that was smart thinking from whichever FG decided to protect her teeth."

TT: Well, it's been another two months and here I am at the same weight, having to wear the same stretchy pants, the same too tight blouses, having the same knee pains, still hiding from cameras, feeling like I've let myself down once again. Something has to give.

FGs: "We don't want to kill her just yet, she is needed in this world by so many, we don't want to cheat them, after all we have to keep her convinced we are her friends. Let's chill on the physical injuries for a while and let's deceive her mind with gimmicks. There are plenty out there, we can keep her occupied for a great amount of time."

TT: (sees a commercial on the television) Immediately, I become desperate and gullible, believing if I chew two delicious gummy bears I will lose 50 pounds in three months. After three months of ingesting weird tasting candy, I am the same size. This cycle continues, shakes, pills, vinegar, shots, patches, teas, red pepper lemonade, fasting, watching "My 600lb Life" for motivation, nothing worked. I am left with less money and more weight! All the weight I did lose, I found in a bag of chips and gained every ounce back. I am not a cheater, so why was I trying to cheat?

FGs: "We are doing so good guys. Look how many days, weeks, months, years that have gone by. All we have to do is keep distracting her and making her subconsciously think she needs us and that she is really comfortable with us. Before we know it, she will just give up and live the rest of her life with us. She is a fighter so we have to remain strong and stubborn. Let's keep filling her head with all the reasons why getting and staying healthy is not right for her. Let's keep discouraging her with thoughts of: "It will take too long to notice a change; it is pointless; let's keep her believing we are part of her DNA makeup and she cannot change us; let's keep her believing that she will never suffer from high blood pressure, diabetes, stroke, or have a heart attack."

"Let's keep convincing her that she is too tired after work to work out, the streets are too dangerous to drive to the gym at 5 a.m. alone, it is too expensive to eat healthy, it takes too much time to prepare healthy meals at home and even if she does, by day three we'll make her tired of leftovers, and let's keep her feeling like she is too busy to fit any exercise in throughout the work day. Once we have control over a person's inner thoughts, the outer words they speak will be of no effect because their actions are controlled by what they truly believe."

I was at my highest weight, 260 pounds. I had convinced myself that I would just be comfortable with it. The FGs can have this battle, I have spent too much time going up and down with them. No one was paying me any attention anyway, so I thought. Until I noticed I was being bullied. My bullying came from love ones, friends, working peers, so it was not obvious until it became undeniable.

A few weeks later I was home meditating again and just like a movie a reel of all the things I hated about having the FGs attached to me played in my mind, clear and in color. I had enough, I imagined myself verbally telling the FGs all the reasons they had to leave me: I am tired of taking the abuse for you guys. You get to hide inside my body, while I have to show my fake smile and show my face to the prejudiced public.

Do people realize the things they say? Fat Genes, you guys are making people around me really expose their ignorance. I hate when people constantly talk about going to the gym whenever I come around, is that supposed to motivate me? Well, it doesn't. The reason it doesn't is because I am distracted by all of your other flaws, like how people brag about being a "vegan" around me but smell like chicken. FGs, you guys have people so uncomfortable they are lying to me for no reason.

Is this their way of suggesting that I become vegan, as if that will help my FGs disappear? How do we make their stupid disappear? I am tired of hearing people who have 10 less Fat Genes me tell me how they can only drink diet Coke because it helps keep them in shape. What shape? A circle! I do believe some people think they are being polite but in actuality they are annoying and ignorant. I was walking up a small flight of stairs, literally five steps, and a lady asked me if I wanted to take the elevator because this may be too much.

No, silly, if it was too much I would not have skipped the elevator. Or when I am at the office carrying a laptop, a note book, a bottle of water, a purse, while wearing heels and I do choose to take the elevator, some nitwit who isn't carrying a thing will come and say, "Oh, I will take the stairs, it is healthier, gets my cardio up." Is that supposed to inspire me? Well, it does not, it makes me want to defend my Fat Genes and hold on to them. I would much rather have Fat Genes than ignorant genes. I am tired of going to gatherings and praying if they have plastic chairs, the kind without arms, because I can barely fit in the ones with arms. They press so hard into my outer thigh I leave with bruises!

I am sick of being in a room full of people and when someone else overweight walks and people peer my way smiling as if to say, you have an equal. I am still annoyed at the time when a larger woman walked into my office and my co-worker sent her to me with the reason being, "I knew you would like her, finally someone larger than you was in the room". I am offended that after every office potluck everyone except me is asked if they want to take leftovers. Are they trying to say, "You don't need anymore"?

I am embarrassed at having to push tables out farther than anyone else's when I go to these Hollywood comedy clubs. They always want to sit me in a booth, knowing I am going to have to push the table all the way out! Our table be the only one sticking out in the row. I have sat and listened to "friends" and colleagues say they would leave their spouse if they ever allowed more than 50 Fat Genes enter their body. They would force their children to run in the heat before they allowed Fat Genes to expose themselves in that child's body, they would starve themselves if they ever thought Fat Genes were coming to them. Then they tell me, "But you are so pretty." Really? You just sat there telling me how you would disrupt your home, abuse your child, and practically kill yourself if you or your family began to look like me but you want me to believe you think I am beautiful? Another case of ignorance.

The good news is, however, with or without you FGs I know I am beautiful. I am intelligent, I am creative, I am successful, and I am a masterpiece and the thoughts of others really do not affect me, I am just tired of hearing it. It saddens me to know there are so many stupid people around me.

I am sick of going to get a Swedish massage and the masseuse thinks he or she needs to apply extra pressure to get through the fat, that mess leaves bruises!!

I am beyond irritated with people telling me I don't need sugar because I will gain more weight. Who are you people and who gave you the right to tell me what I should not eat? Meanwhile, you standing with a duck gut and eating sugar while staring at me. You are a joke to me, but if I say that out loud it will come across as the big girl is angry again.

I am frustrated with people thinking giving me food makes for a friendly gesture. I am embarrassed that people think they should order extra food because I am coming.
I understand most people are not aware of their own ignorance so I let it slide. I am tired of allowing ignorance to slide!

I am offended and hurt that people equate size with being mean or having an attitude. I walk in their rooms with a pleasant attitude and smile but still people immediately become uncomfortable and start acting like since I am large, I must be in charge so they scatter away or, worse, they come over and ask why am I angry? WHAT? I am as happy as a lark, why do people equate bigger with angry? I am tired of it!

I am outraged that people want to talk over my food while I am eating, then when I ask them to not stand over me while I am sitting and eating, they have the nerve to say she is serious about her food, leave her alone. No, you are annoying, I am eating a meal and you are literally standing over me, talking and spitting with every "P" word on top of my food! This has nothing to do with weight or loving food!

I am tired of having to only wear stretchy clothes because button-up pants make me feel as if I am being sawed in half. I am tired of paying a higher price because I need a size XXL shirt. I am sad that my knees and back are starting to hurt when I stand or go down stairs. I am not taking the hit for your guys anymore.

TT: After all these years, I truly believed you guys were with me to comfort me. I knew at times you made me feel a bit uncomfortable but for the most part you made me feel fulfilled. We have to part ways. The doctor has given me a fair warning.
FGs: Wow, TT, we never imagined you to be so gullible. We have been with you for over forty years and you are ready to dismiss us after hearing fifteen minutes of "lies" from a man wearing a white coat. How dare you think of disregarding us completely? Who was with you when were afraid, who comforted you during your divorce, who guided you to delicious sweets and sat with you at the end of your stressful work days? It was us that cried with you, worried with you, when you were unsure about your ability to successfully raise your daughter. We maintained your sanity when you wanted to lose your mind! Days you wanted to give up on everything, we convinced you to have a great meal, sleep it off and live to eat another day!
TT: The man in the white coat has a medical degree and he is telling the truth. I have heard about how you guys creep up and destroy people. You guys are best friends with the silent killers, heart attack and strokes. I refuse to allow you to take me out. You have to go, you are trying to kill me!
FGs: Well now you are saying you want to kill us! How does that make you better than us?
TT: I am killing you to live and fulfill my purpose in life.

FGs: So here we are. Let the games begin.
TT: This is not a game, this is my life...

Chapter Eight

Loser Mentality

Finding my Worth

I finally had to stop communicating with the FGs and talk honestly with myself. I questioned myself, asking how many Saturdays was I going to spend locked in the house watching "My 600lb Life" marathons while eating pizza, chips, popcorn, nachos, washing it all down with soda? What kind of twisted, sick-mind-warp had I allowed the FGs to put in my brain?

How long was I going to say single moms deserve extra treats because we do the work of two, and allow my treat to be edible? I do deserve to treat myself but instead of running to purchase $4 munchie meals and $6 extra-sweet coffees, save the money and allow it to add up until I have enough for a Gucci purse. How long was I going to stay at a corporate job filled with stress, taking each project personal, being underpaid, overworked, being unappreciated, then accepting office pizza parties as a peace offering? How much was I going to eat before I realized I was living in a vicious cycle of me trying to fill a bottomless pit of empty emotions with food, and to no avail?

How long was I going to hold on to the beliefs I had embedded in my brain telling me that I am to eat at eating time, eat everything on my plate, and eat whatever is served to me? How long was I going to defeat myself by saying being a single mom was too tough and eating snacks would relieve some of the burden? How much longer would I feed into the FGs' deception and give them credit for my failure? Treating them as if they are stronger than my will power!

When was I going to stop the bunch of madness that the FGs had set in motion with their distractions? In 2016, my cousin Sean passed away. He also fought with FGs, and unfortunately he lost. He was over 600lb when he died. Losing him right after Darrin were two of the greatest blows to my life. I literally felt a piece of me leave and go with each of them. Losing them back-to-back made me feel like I had no chance to grieve or deal with challenges, I just had to keep moving. All that suppression made me eat. What was it going to take for me to release guilt and know it is not my moral obligation to eat everything and accept that eating never really helped the pain anyway?

How long before I acknowledged that all this time I'd been sleeping with the enemy! Me, I am my own worst enemy. My enemies literally live under my own skin. Although people hurt my feelings, played a part in molding my thought process, called me names, sabotaged my work, talked behind my back, cheated on me, when it came to acting against my success, it was all me.

When was I going to break the habit of saying I do everything alone. I need a workout buddy, I need a nutritionist. When was I going to stop saying I know God will never leave me alone or forsake me, but still complain about being all alone? I had everything I needed within myself. What I didn't know, I could Google.

How many more times was I going to trick myself by saying all I need is some motivation? Then spending a ton of money on new workout clothes, pills, shakes, gummies, creams, detox potions, shrinking teas, and drops all because they would "motivate" me to lose the FGs and become healthy? My doctor offered me bariatric surgery. I am thankful I had enough sense to know nothing was going to help me become healthy until I got emotionally fit first.

How long was I going to say leaving the house at 5 a.m. to go to a gym was too dangerous, too cold, too dark, when there have been days that I have left to catch a flight that early and I see several elderly people out walking in peace around my neighborhood? How many more times would I say, I will start on Monday after work, knowing that particular Monday had not come in years? The best day to start is today!

When was I going to stop being a victim and realize I had been living captive to the FGs for years?

Under my own command. When was I going to live a healthy lifestyle and be an example to my daughter, my nieces and nephews? They see my drive and my success but were they seeing me love me? Was I showing them how to love themselves? How long was I going to disrespect the temple that was given to me to walk this Earth in? The very temple I invited Jesus to dwell in? Where does He fit with so much clutter going on?

These enemies are much bigger than us, if we build them up in our belief as such. I made my FGs so huge I could not face them alone or with my own power. I have to call on Jesus and trust that He alone will sustain me. I have to do all I can, then stand. If I claim that "greater is He that is in me, than he that is in the world, why am I allowing evil, damaging thoughts to rule my world and beat me up? After asking myself these questions and more I concluded and walked away with enlightenment and awareness of my daily energies, the level of vibration I dwell in and what I allow to influence my thinking. I am no longer under the spell of the FGs.

I have learned to use discernment when people speak and know when they are speaking from their own insecurities or being a real friend who is giving good advice or sharing wisdom. I am blessed to have my friend Steve, who introduced me to the world of meditation. I have been able to discover the lack of success has been self-inflicted. I am thankful for my friend Hawk. Because of him, I have learned to really listen to my own body. Although Hawk was not gifted with FGs, he did suffer a stroke at the age of 34 and did not listen immediately to his body. Thank God he is fully recovered today. His lesson to listen and his testimony has taught me a lot.

Then there is my sister-friend, Keesha, who is my personal, healthy lifestyle advocate who reminds me that a healthy lifestyle provides an opportunity of quality wealth, free will to invest in yourself, discipline to change and faith to see the impossible. I know that I am not alone and I have these three and a host of others rooting for me. The positive energy from them outweighs the FGs any day. It is just up to me to take action and do right by myself. To top all of that, I have the greatest source of energy and power of all. We all need a great power. You can choose who you like, but I chose the only God I know, I call Him Jesus. I can only do what works for me. I have everything I need, I have had it for years, now is the time to use it.

I knew this journey for me this was not going to be an overnight success. The FGs did not appear overnight so I had to accept they would not leave overnight. I have to pace myself, taking it slow and steady. I must utilize the same discipline I use for work and clients. I need to learn to love working out and appreciate the natural high it leaves me with after every session, a high that is better than any energy I have ever had. I have to take on a loser mentality and lose the self-inflicted negativity, lose the weight (FGs), lose the low self-esteem, lose the self-doubt, and lose that mediocre acceptance.

As you read this book, ask yourself, what is holding you back from gaining your absolute freedom? My worst enemies were my FGs and me giving them the ability to blind me to myself. These enemies are quite creative. Even with me being aware of them. acknowledging them, and fighting with them, I know now that I cannot fight them alone. After my success of losing 60 of them, they found an even better way to deceive me and trick me into letting them return again with friends. What is your worst enemy? I now accept and know my value and worth and absolutely refuse to lower for anyone, not even myself.

Chapter Nine

In Tune with My Body Needs

I wish I could start this chapter off by announcing that the battle of the bulge is over. I have successfully killed the FGs and can now rest. I wish that was the conclusion, but it is not. The reality is, unlike the FGs, which are a figment of my imagination, my being overweight and unhealthy is real and will be a life-long struggle. In this chapter of my life I am more aware of what I allow to distract me. I am more in tune with what my body actually needs. I now make time for me and at first it was a shocker or maybe hurtful to some people. Normally, I skip me and do them, so putting me first was scary but I had to be true to me, I have to save me, I have to destroy the FGs before they destroy me.

When I first shared this book with my publisher, he required me to share more of my story. It scared me because I was afraid that I would hurt people's feelings or come off as bitter. One of the biggest misconceptions I had was thinking if I admitted some of the beliefs I had instilled in me were not right for me, it would be like saying my grandmother, father and mother were wrong. I would never say that because in my mind these three people are as close to perfect as you can get. I know there was no ill intent ever, but some of their words did indeed warp my mindset and hurt my feelings. I can admit now that some of the things they taught me did not work well for me, personally, and now as an adult I have the power to change them.

I know all of their teachings and words came from a good place and were filled with love, so I did not want to be misunderstood. The FGs wanted me to stay silent but because I am finally taking care of me and I said no, I must share my journey. I took the advice of LaVal, my publisher. I dug deep and shared it all. The end result is I feel great! This writing process has helped me more than I anticipated and it for sure jumpstarted my journey to health. Just like the FGs came in groups, I had to attack them in groups and let each of them know I no longer trust you. Over the years, it seems as if they formed cliques and throughout the day, they would take shifts to work on my mind and control me, resulting in their gains and my loss. The groups are:

Team Stress: The FGs had my body but decided to get greedy and attack my soul. I said I trust God but I was still carrying burdens. I had so many little things that I was carrying and one day it just clicked. I no longer stress over the lady driving slow with her blinker on for 2 miles when I am rushing to work. I no longer stress over the co-worker who does not speak back to me. I can leave early to be on time but if the kid walking to school is playing in the street and makes me one minute late, I can't stress over not being Jesus and perfect every day for work. I cannot stress over why my neighbor insist on parking his car in front of my house and he has a garage the same as I. I cannot stress over who our current state leader is.

I cannot stress over why my ex-husband decided to leave my daughter and me and remarry a lady with a daughter and care for them as if they were the originals. I cannot stress over who thinks I am acting bougie because I don't like talking loud in public.

I cannot stress over who is offended by my respectful decline to attend a 9 p.m. event on a weeknight. I gave all of that up.

Team Anger: I cannot fix stupid, so I don't even acknowledge anymore. Growing up, the word stupid was not allowed to be said in our household. I still will never call anyone with a learning disability or someone taking a longer time to learn a new lesson that word.

However, as an adult, there are some people who know better, they know they know better and I know they know better, yet they still do things out of line. They are stupid.

For example, I could be sitting in a church pew that is built to seat 10 "standard size" adults, but it feels like 13 of us are on the row because the usher saw fit to squeeze a few slightly larger adults in a row, then comes "Sister, I am late on purpose so the congregation can see my new outfit. I have to sit in that row because the camera is positioned to start filming there first", and she demands to sit in the same already at-capacity row, and because she may have a nice shape or her "fancy clothes" look appealing, people, especially the men, try to scoot over and make room for her.

Ma'am, you will not fit! Please go sit in the back row that is empty and come to church early. Heck, at least show up on time next week and sit here. You, my dear, are stupid. Sir, you in the Sears suit, she will NOT fit, so stop trying to scoot. If you want "Sister Shake 'Em Up" to sit here, be a man, get up and give her your seat. Sir, you are stupid!

I would get so angry, I would be the one to move. My efforts at being on time became irrelevant. I arrived on time to be in the sanctuary, otherwise sitting in the back row or in the balcony for me at times would be distracting because that is where all the late comers went. The first half of service would be filled with constant movement, talking and seat arranging. Then there is the option of going to the overflow room and watching on television, but I can stay home in bed if I want to watch a service on television.

The whole experience would ruin moments of my praise and worship. Instead of completely focusing on the Lord, I would be thinking of other things, like, Sunday dinner. That made me feel stupid and bloated. Had to let it go. If I cannot control it, if it does not jeopardize my health or my freedom, I simply don't care.

It seems as if it was instant. When I learned to focus and have more control over my anger and stress, my pants got looser and my shoulders felt lighter. I was not feeding those groups of FGs what they needed to trigger my snacking and they quickly went away. I noticed my stomach was not as bloated, which taught me, just like the empty air that was contained in my body, the anger and stress were empty emotions filled with air that were very unnecessary. I confronted these two groups first because they report directly to strokes and heart attacks and they were on the fast track to kill me. The rest of the groups are causing me to have more patience and be a bit more creative when it comes to killing them.

Team Comfort: These guys hate to feel sore after a workout, they filled my head with thoughts of, "You won't be able to go up the stairs at work", "It will hurt to lift your arms and work on your computer", "It will not feel good when you walk. You are too far out of shape, you may break something if you try to workout. Sleep in, the bed is super warm and comfortable. Have a seat and watch television, you have worked hard all day and deserve a break". I knew I could succeed at relaxing, what if I failed at working out? Why break out of my comfort zone and chance wasting time?

I had reminded myself that working is in my DNA. I've worked since I was 15 years old. I have worked many years making corporations more wealthy. I have worked for clients, making sure they succeed. I worked harder when I knew the chances of the outcome would be a fail. I became immune to the many "no" answers I received when I pitched something for my clients, but I kept working. Eventually, some of my expected "no's" became a "yes". I accepted and succeeded completing work for corporate offices that were not in my job description. I took myself out of my comfort zone and did the work.

Some of the times, I really did not want to do the work for others. I always want everyone to succeed, but truth be told, some days I just did not feel like waking up early to make a phone call to the East Coast. I did not feel like staying up late drafting a press release. I did not feel like working overtime to make sure a doctor could print a prescription when he came into his office in the morning. I did not want to do it, but I did it all without one verbal complaint. I did it and I did it well. I asked myself, why didn't I look at working on myself the same way? My mindset had to changed.

I now refuse to start my weekday without a workout. My intent is to wake up at 5 a.m. and go to the gym. If I don’t make it, I have to not beat myself up over it and take advantage of the way my body is set to automatically wake up at 6 a.m. no matter what. Instead of lying in bed watching television, or catching up on the latest social media news, I get up and go to my in-house treadmill or I log onto my Estrada Fitness

Program online and get in a quick 30-minute workout. I have to do this for me. I have to want me to succeed as much as I want others to succeed.

Team Independently Lazy: I don't like housework, I don't like dusting, mopping, vacuuming, sweeping, none of it. I never liked it and probably never will, but I always get it done. As the middle child, I was often forced to do most of the housework alone because the "bigs" were either at an outside job or they had already married and moved away. The "smalls" were too young, or if they did try to help they made a bigger mess to clean. I was forced to do it and I got it done. As a single mom, I just wanted the work done, so I maintained the house alone. Just like the "smalls" when I would give my daughter a chore, it took her all day and I just wanted it to be over.

Team Independently Lazy convinced me that working out and eating healthy were chores and I would feel drained before I even started. The FGs told me that I had the power to decline these chores. Unlike housework, where mother would dictate my efforts, or as an adult having to maintain home cleanliness for the sake of hygiene, I could decline the chore of healthy eating and eat what came easy, and I could decline going to the gym or waking up early to work out because I technically don't have to do this.

There would be no one to punish me for not doing this work. I no longer look at eating healthy or working out as a chore, I look at it as a blessing and a gift to honor my temple by taking care of it. Just like having a clean house is a good look, having a healthy body is a good look and being healthy comes with far more benefits. I am also gifted with not having to do this part of my journey alone. I have met new friends that are into fitness so watching them encourages me to workout. Even if they quit, I will continue, but for now, it is a good motivator.

As far as eating healthy, my daughter is a culinary student who still lives with me. She has taken it upon herself to do some of the cooking, which is always healthy, and she shops for the groceries because she has done the schoolwork and has learned about healthy eating. She keeps me stocked with healthy snacks. In fact, as I was writing this chapter, she walked into my office and left a bowl of cut-up Cara Cara oranges, organic strawberries, grapes and passion fruit. Looking at food and exercise is no longer a chore to me, it is a privilege and I am blessed to have a small team around me that I am finally allowing to help!

Team Lust; These FGs come with consequences, but I have to get through them. Normally, when someone mentions the word lust, we think of a sinful physical attraction to another human being. Not me. My lust was not for men but rather for food. The thought of a good meal made my heart flutter. Knowing I was going out to dinner and they would serve super-sized portions of high caloric food brought me so much joy.

I would daydream about the meal. I would crave the feeling of an ice -old energy drink in my hand. I could taste the sugar in the drink just by thinking about it. I would get pleasurable chills when I heard ice filling a glass and a sugary drink being poured.

Hearing the ruffling of a chip bag was a huge turn-on. That noise could silence out any distraction around. It was ridiculous and we had to finally break up. I had to face the fact that I was using junk to fulfill a desire I had to be loved. I had to tell these FGs that never again could I trust them and never again could they use my body as their home. I welcomed them in and they made me a prisoner in my own body. When I stop feeding them what they want, they put up a big fight! They caused me withdrawals, which included headaches, jitters, sadness, anger and frustration. This team is also quite jealous. I will be honest, I have not completely cut out junk food, but I have made big changes. I still drink my coffee in the morning, but now I do not add flavored creamer AND 10 sugar packets. I only use the flavored creamer.

I no longer eat the big family-size bag of chips, I will get the small, three for $.99 bag and only eat one bag and my limit is once a week. I no longer eat a huge bowl of ice cream, I eat a couple of teaspoons and call it quits. That is only if I have ice cream. Most times I just bypass it altogether. Even with me still having some junk, the FGs are not happy. They constantly want more but I have to remain strong and overpower them with the fact, if I can't handle a little, I won't have any. This group continues to be my biggest foe.

Team All Talk: One thing I cannot stand is a talker. "I am about to", "I used to", "One day"... Stop talking about it and be about it. I despise when people throw out false promises. I would much rather not talk at all. In fact, if a person comes at me too many times with unfulfilled words, I will cut them out of my life. I have no problem blocking phone numbers, ignoring emails, or walking into a room and completely not seeing you on purpose. I cannot stand a fraud! I will lovingly accept you for all that you cannot do before I will continue to entertain you and your make-believe promises. In return, I make it my life to keep my word to others. If I cannot do something, I will not leave you with false hope. The answer is simply no. I would hate to leave someone in limbo, waiting on me, knowing I cannot help or I would not give my best energy to fulfill.

It is easier to just say no up front, this gives the other person time to seek other resources. This is a demand I put on people, and on myself regarding other people. If it is not baseball or basketball, I don't like games! I don't even like card games, so why was I playing games with myself? I had to hold myself to the same standards when it came to me dealing with me. When I have thoughts of skipping a workout, I tell myself, "You are all talk, no action". When find myself on a repeated trip to a fast food place, I remind myself that a healthy body will remain a daydream if I just talk about healthy eating. I have to create my own reality and that takes action.

Team Boredom: This is the most deceiving group of FGs. I am a single mother who works two full-time jobs, chose to advance my freelance writing into a book, have parents who still like to be active but not necessarily drive as much, have vacant walls in my house that need pictures hanging and paint, I have shelves of unread books, I have closets of clothes I need to go through. I have friends that I text but never call. I have friends and family that I have not spoken to in months that I could call or, better yet, visit.

When do I have time and why do I get bored? If that is not the most foolish thing, I don't know what is. I was allowing this team to control my mind with thoughts of I have nothing "fun" to do or "That is going to be too tiring, you deserve a break" or, "You spent all day talking at work, take this time to be quiet", only to leave me sitting on the sofa, eating and mindlessly watching television.

I made a list of things that I need to do or can do, and when I think I am bored, I pull out my list. If I indeed do not feel like working around the house or writing, because I do get writer's block, I put on a song and dance alone. This always cracks me up because I am not a dancer. Just seeing me trying to move like a Soul Train dancer is hilarious. The point is, I find something to do. Sitting idle is only for when I need rest. If I have enough energy to think I am bored and eat snacks, I have enough energy to get up and move, even if it is just to the corner and back!

Team Guilt: I am not my failures! I am not the Christ! This is a phase. I had to embed that in my head and make myself believe and accept. I am all about success! I am all about completion! So when I had two failed marriages, lost a home, did not book a client on a major show, did not book a client to be on the cover of a magazine, did not stop the doctor's computer from running slowly, I felt like a failure.

When did not prevent my friend's daughter from being molested, did not stop cancer from killing my friend's mother, did not stop cancer from attacking my own mother, did not save my cousins from dying, did not obtain a promotion in corporate work, did not get my friends and family hired at my corporate job, the FGs told me I had let everyone down.

I felt like there should have been something I could have done and I messed up. Today, I know that in all cases, I did all that I could to succeed. The cases that I absolutely could not control, I did all I could to help make the painful process less stressful. I was looking for validation from outside sources. This validation would have come when I booked every show, when I remained married, when I cured cancer. I placed ridiculous expectations on myself that were beyond my control and, quite frankly, no one held me accountable for. I had to learn to validate myself. I am satisfied with whatever the outcome is after I have given my all and done all I could possibly do to achieve success. If the answer is still no, then it is just no. Tomorrow is a brand-new day.

Working to murder these personal groups and thought-processes that I have allowed to run my world, I have uncovered so many layers of untruths I gave power to. Writing this book has been my necessary therapy that was long overdue for me.

I am sure there are more groups dwelling within me that I have not tapped into. The difference is, now I am aware and I am prepared for them. I am watchful of myself.

This book purposely did not contain a bunch of statistics or horror stories. I said in the beginning sometimes you have to laugh at yourself. We need to lighten up. Reading a bunch of scary numbers or research about how you will have a heart attack tonight will add stress and sometimes we need a break from stress. I believe there is a lesson in everything, even if we are laughing while we are learning.

We all will face challenges in some shape or form. I personally have experienced, have dealt with and gone THROUGH two divorces, child molestation, being conned out of money, death of very close friends and family members, people lying to my face, domestic (mental) abuse, being laid off a job, busted investments, being judged, losing a home, ill parents, being a single mother, being the only income, baby daddy skipping out on child support and not active in my child's life, people hating me for no reason, waste of time boyfriends, being engaged to a man that left town and married someone else, being treated like I was unworthy by the church, jobs that treat employees like numbers and not humans.... *whew,* I have been through some crap and that is exactly what it was - CRAP - and I did exactly what I said I did, I went THROUGH it.

No matter what you have gone through or are currently going through, please don't let it be your reason to create excuses to stand still or lose focus on what your purpose in life is. I have made it, and every day I remind myself that I am in a constant battle, I am not my past, I am not my circumstance, I am not my failures, I am not destined to fail. I am powerful, I am wise, I am surrounded by greatness, I am gorgeous, I am in control! I encourage you to do the same.

Although I've had fun with making my Fat Genes into make-believe, cartoon characters, the reality is there are truly evil adversaries that exist and dwell among us to set up stumbling blocks to stop us from achieving greatness! I did not recognize how active they were in contributing to my self-sabotaging until I wrote them down and kept thinking back to the core of things and asking myself, "Why"?

We all live in a fast-paced world, things happen to us and we barely have time to process it before we move on to the next crisis. We have to find time to download all of this stuff and process it all. Otherwise, I learned in writing this book, I am capable of just moving with the flow and opening doors for defeat to overtake me. So many us are dying at a young age. In my peer group alone, it seems as if 40 is the new 90! We are dying from stress (hearts giving out, strokes), diabetes, aneurysms, cancer, things that as children we expected our grandparents to die from.

Writing this book was my eye opener. I am aware of triggers that come to attack me. Perhaps writing a book may be your gateway also. Whatever it takes for you, don't be deceived, do not be afraid to confront the root of your self-sabotage, and certainly don't be too lazy to expose your adversaries because they are never lazy, they stay up working! The reality of my story is, my FGs are really just my own ego. It has only been a short time since I came to terms with this. My ego was causing me to resist my own greatness. Now that I am aware and know when to shut the FGs, my ego down, I find myself happier than I have been in a very long time. I have more natural energy and I am attracting so many positive people and opportunities. I am choosing healthy on purpose and it feels wonderful! This new outlook was the start of the best chapter of my life and I know each chapter moving forward will only get better.

The end, or shall I say, my beginning...

For speaking engagements, seminars, books signings, contact:
Email: tcpr4u@yahoo.com
Instagram: CarmouchePR
Facebook: facebook.com/tcarmouche1

Made in the USA
Las Vegas, NV
15 August 2024

93899007R00089